BIOELECTRONICS AND MEDICAL DEVICES

Applications and Technology

BIOELECTRONICS AND MEDICAL DEVICES

Applications and Technology

Edited by

Garima Srivastava, PhD

Manju Khari, PhD

AAP | APPLE ACADEMIC PRESS

First edition published 2022

Apple Academic Press Inc.
1265 Goldenrod Circle, NE,
Palm Bay, FL 32905 USA

4164 Lakeshore Road, Burlington,
ON, L7L 1A4 Canada

CRC Press
6000 Broken Sound Parkway NW,
Suite 300, Boca Raton, FL 33487-2742 USA

2 Park Square, Milton Park,
Abingdon, Oxon, OX14 4RN UK

Library and Archives Canada Cataloguing in Publication

Title: Bioelectronics and medical devices : applications and technology / edited by Garima Srivastava, PhD, Manju Khari, PhD.

Names: Srivastava, Garima, 1976- editor. | Khari, Manju, editor.

Description: Includes bibliographical references and index.

Identifiers: Canadiana (print) 20200360477 | Canadiana (ebook) 20200360531 | ISBN 9781771889230 (hardcover) | ISBN 9781774638088 (softcover) | ISBN 9781003054405 (ebook)

Subjects: LCSH: Medical electronics. | LCSH: Medical instruments and apparatus.

Classification: LCC R856 .B56 2021 | DDC 610.28—dc23

Library of Congress Cataloging-in-Publication Data

Names: Srivastava, Garima, 1976- editor. | Khari, Manju, editor.

Title: Bioelectronics and medical devices : applications and technology / edited by Garima Srivastava, Manju Khari.

Description: First edition. | Palm Bay : Apple Academic Press, 2021. | Includes bibliographical references and index. | Summary: "Bioelectronics and Medical Devices: Applications and Technology provides an abundance of information on new applications being used today for biomedical applications. The book covers a wide range of concepts and technologies used in biomedical applications, discussing such modern technological methods as the Internet of Things, e-pills, biomedical sensors, support vector machines, wireless devices, image and signal processing in e-health, and machine learning. It also discusses the different types of antennas, including antennas using RF energy harvesting for biomedical applications. This book contains three chapters on the various kinds of antennas used for biomedical applications, which make this book unique as this information is not generally discussed in the field of biomedical engineering. It also includes a discussion on software implementation for the devices used in biomedical applications, of course. Key features: Provides in-depth information on the major topics in real-life biomedical applications. Considers both theoretical as well as experimental approaches Topics include: The Internet of Things for health care and monitoring Antennas for biomedical applications using RF energy harvesting Biomedical sensors Software fault proneness with support vector machine biomedical applications Image and signal processing in e-health applications E-pill for biomedical applications Machine learning implementation in bioinformatics This book will be valuable for undergraduate, postgraduate, and PhD students working in the biomedical application field. It will also be beneficial for scientists and medical professionals who are interested in the latest biomedical technologies being used today"-- Provided by publisher.

Identifiers: LCCN 2020046150 (print) | LCCN 2020046151 (ebook) | ISBN 9781771889230 (hardcover) | ISBN 9781774638088 (softcover) | ISBN 9781003054405 (ebook)

Subjects: MESH: Electronics, Medical--instrumentation | Equipment and Supplies | Biosensing Techniques--instrumentation | Biomedical Technology--instrumentation

Classification: LCC R855.3 (print) | LCC R855.3 (ebook) | NLM QT 26 | DDC 610.285--dc23

LC record available at https://lccn.loc.gov/2020046150

LC ebook record available at https://lccn.loc.gov/2020046151

ISBN: 978-1-77188-923-0 (hbk)
ISBN: 978-1-77463-808-8 (pbk)
ISBN: 978-1-00305-440-5 (ebk)

About the Editors

Garima Srivastava, PhD

Assistant Professor, Ambedkar Institute of Advanced Communication Technologies and Research, Government of India National Capital Territory, Delhi, India

Garima Srivastava, PhD, is an Assistant Professor at Ambedkar Institute of Advanced Communication Technologies and Research, under the Govt. of NCT Delhi, India. She has more than 15 years of teaching experience. Her areas of interest include wireless communication, MIMO technologies, internet of things, microstrip antennas, UWB antennas, and reconfigurable and circular polarized antennas. She has more than 25 published papers in refereed national and international journals published by IEEE, ACM, Springer, Inderscience, and Elsevier), and has presented at many conferences. She has chaired many IEEE conferences and organized different workshops in area of Rf and icrowave. She has also been the technical program committee member of various IEEE international conferences and journals. She also delivers expert talks at various institutions at conferences. She has authored a book chapter on topic smart antennas. She holds her PhD in Electronics and Communication Engineering and a master's degree in electronics engineering from the University of Allahabad, India.

Manju Khari, PhD

Assistant Professor, Ambedkar Institute of Advanced Communication Technologies and Research, under the Government of India National Capital Territory, Delhi, India

Manju Khari, PhD, is an Assistant Professor at the Ambedkar Institute of Advanced Communication Technologies and Research, under the Government of India National Capital Territory, Delhi, India, affiliated with Guru Gobind Singh Indraprastha University, Delhi, India. Her research interests are software testing, software quality, software metrics, information security, optimization, and nature-inspired algorithm. She has 70 published papers in refereed national and international journals and conferences, such as IEEE,

ACM, Springer, Inderscience, and Elsevier, and six book chapters with Springer. She is also co-author of two books published by the National Council of Educational Research and Training.

She has delivered an expert talk and guest lectures at international conferences and is a member of the technical program committee of an international conference in Hyderabad, India. She is also a life member of several international and national research societies. In addition, she is associated with much international publishers and is a guest editor of the *International Journal of Advanced Intelligence Paradigms,* reviewer for the *International Journal of Forensic Engineering,* and an editorial board member of the *International Journal of Software Engineering and Knowledge Engineering.*

Dr. Khari holds a PhD in Computer Science and Engineering from the National Institute of Technology Patna, India, and received her master's degree in Information Security from the Ambedkar Institute of Advanced Communication Technology and Research, formerly known as Ambedkar Institute of Technology, affiliated with Guru Gobind Singh Indraprastha University, Delhi, India..

Contents

Contributors

Sarita Ahlawat
Ambedkar Institute of Advanced Communication Technologies and Research, Delhi–110031, India, E-mail: saritaahlawat4@gmail.com

Sushmita Bhushan
Department of ECE, Ambedkar Institute of Advanced Communication Technologies and Research, Delhi, India, E-mail: Sushmita.iert@gmail.com

Dimple Chandra
Assistant Professor, Computer Science and Engineering Department, NIET, Greater Noida, Uttar Pradesh, India, E-mail: dimplechandra1988@gmail.com

Renu Dalal
Assistant Professor, Computer Science and Engineering Department, AIACT&R, GGSIPU, Delhi, India, E-mail: dalalrenu1987@gmail.com

Binod Kumar Kanaujia
School of Computational and Integrative Sciences, Jawaharlal Nehru University, New Delhi–110067, India, E-mail: bkkanaujia@ieee.org

Manju Khari
Assistant Professor, Computer Science and Engineering Department, Ambedkar Institute of Advanced Communication Technologies and Research, GGSIPU, Geeta Colony, Delhi–110031, India, E-mail: manjukhari@yahoo.co.in

Sachin Kumar
School of Electronics Engineering, Kyungpook National University, Daegu–41566, Republic of Korea; Department of Electronics and Communication Engineering, SRM Institute of Science and Technology, Chennai – 603203, India, E-mail: gupta.sachin0708@gmail.com

Sanjeev Kumar
Department of ECE, Ambedkar Institute of Advanced Communication Technologies and Research, Delhi, India, E-mail: skgaale@gmail.com

Deepti Mishra
Associate Professor, G. L. Bajaj Institute of Technology and Management, Greater Noida, India, E-mail: itsdeepti.s@gmail.com

Sandeep Kumar Palaniswamy
Department of Electronics and Communication Engineering, SRM Institute of Science and Technology, Chennai–603203, India

Divya Prakash Pattanayak
MTech Student, Department of Electronics and Communication, Ambedkar Institute of Advanced Communication Technologies and Research, New Delhi, India

Surya Prakash Pattanayak
MTech Student, Department of Electronics and Communication,
Ambedkar Institute of Advanced Communication Technologies and Research, New Delhi, India,
E-mail: suryankbabu@gmail.com

Thipparaju Rama Rao
Department of Electronics and Communication Engineering,
SRM Institute of Science and Technology, Chennai–603203, India

Shobhit Saxena
Department of Electronics Engineering, Indian Institute of Technology (Indian School of Mines),
Dhanbad–826004, India

Shailesh
Ambedkar Institute of Advanced Communication Technologies and Research, Delhi–110031, India,
E-mail: shailesh.jayant404@gmail.com

Ajay Sharma
Associate Professor, Department of Electronics and Communication Engineering,
United College of Engineering and Research, Naini, Prayagraj, Uttar Pradesh–211010, India,
E-mail: ajaysharma.ucer@gmail.com

Shikhar Sharma
Ambedkar Institute of Advanced Communication Technologies and Research, Geeta Colony,
Delhi–110031, India

Hanuman Prasad Shukla
Professor, Department of Electronics and Communication Engineering,
United College of Engineering and Research, Naini, Prayagraj, Uttar Pradesh–211010, India,
E-mail: hpshukla@united.ac.in

Neeta Singh
Ambedkar Institute of Advanced Communication Technologies and Research, Delhi–110031, India,
E-mail: neeta.singh90@gmail.com

Garima Srivastava
Department of Electronics and Communication Engineering,
Ambedkar Institute of Advanced Communication Technologies and Research, Delhi–110031, India,
E-mail: garima.shrivastav@aiactr.ac

Abbreviations

ACPA	aperture-coupled patch antenna
ADC	analog to digital converter
AM	amplitude modulation
AR	axial ratio
ASA	annular slot antennas
BR	branch
CAD	computer-aided detection
CP	circularly polarized
CPW	coplanar waveguide
CT	computed tomography
DBS	direct broadcasting services
DFR	transform reconstruction technique
DG	diversity gain
DGS	defected ground structure
DoA	direction of arrival
DSP	digital signal processor
DSRR	double split-ring resonator
DT	decision tree
EBG	electromagnetic band-gap
ECC	electronic communications committee
EEG	electroencephalogram
EM	electromagnetic
FCC	Federal Communications Commission
FN	false negative
FP	false positive
FSS	frequency selective surfaces
GB	gradient boosted
GERD	gastrointestinal reflux disease
GI	gastrointestinal
GSGSG	ground-signal-ground-signal-ground
ICTs	information and communication technologies
INAIL	National Institute for Insurance Against Accidents at Work
IOMT	internet of medical things

IoT	internet of things
ISM	industrial, scientific, and medical
KHARE	Kinect Hololens Assisted Rehabilitation Experience
KNN	K nearest neighbors
L	level
LCP	liquid crystalline polymer
LHCP	left hand circularly polarized
LOC	line of code
MDP	metrics data program
MICS	medical implant communications systems
MIMO	multiple input multiple output
ML	machine learning
MRI	magnetic resonance imaging
MSP	medical signal processing
PBG	photonic bandgap
PDMS	poly-dimethylsiloxane
PIFA	planar inverted F antenna
PZT	lead zirconate titanite
RBF	radial basis function
RF	random forests
RFI	radio frequency interference
RHCP	right hand circularly polarized
SAR	specific absorption rate
SFPP	software fault proneness prediction
SRR	split-ring resonators
sSRR	symmetric SRR
SVM	support vector machine
TN	true negative
TP	true positive
UHF	ultra-high frequencies
UWB	ultra-wideband
WBAN	wireless body area networks
WiMAX	worldwide interoperability for microwave access
WLAN	wireless local area network
WMTS	wireless medical telemetry service
WPAN	wireless personal area networks
ZOR	zeroth-order resonance

Preface

This book provides fundamental information that can be used by undergraduate, postgraduate, and PhD students working in the biomedical field. The book is also beneficial for scientists and doctors who are interested in the latest technologies being used in the biomedical field. The objective of the book is to guide readers about different biomedical applications being used. It also gives a brief overview of how health care is related to the internet of things. Image and signal processing is also explained, and its application in health care are discussed.

Machine learning (ML) and its relation to bioinformatics are explained. All the concepts are well explained with the help of appropriate illustrations and examples. The analysis, presentation, and physical interpretation of theory are purposefully lucid to ensure that students are able to grasp the subject with ease. Key equations and formulas have been highlighted. The book also includes discussion, software implementation, and hardware of the devices used for biomedical applications.

CHAPTER 1

Internet of Things for Health Care and Health Monitoring

DEEPTI MISHRA

Associate Professor, G. L. Bajaj Institute of Technology and Management, Greater Noida, India, E-mail: itsdeepti.s@gmail.com

ABSTRACT

Internet of things (IoT)-empowered devices allow patients and users to handle health care issues and are more beneficial for health monitoring by offering better fitness. IoT provides a lot of valuable prospects in the domain of medicine. As health care-related services are expensive, such IoT devices related to health care are very much utilized by the people and these are grasping their roots very rapidly. The medical devices can gather worthy information regarding users' symptoms for the disease and when associated with the internet they provide real-time monitoring of symptoms. Health care devices with the internet can support remote care as patients can more regulate their treatments when they are aware of the complications regularly in an easy manner. There are many ways of applying IoT in medical devices such as wearables fitness bands for monitoring heart rates, walk steps, blood pressure so that patients can be given personalized care, etc. A continuous glucose monitor is a medical device enabled with IoT and is used to uninterruptedly monitor the glucose level of diabetic patients. The chapter presents the concept, functioning, and applications of IoT on various biomedical devices for health care and health monitoring for both patients and physicians.

1.1 INTRODUCTION

The internet of things (IoT) is a broad system of devices that can communicate, share, and transfer the data digitally in real-time with complete security via the internet. It means devices are capable enough for retrieval and transmission of information using a communication channel. Let us assume an example, we can read books, newspapers, and search jobs in any domain when we connect to the internet. All the information is not stored at the same location, but the mobile searches the keywords and displays in a single search. IoT applies heterogeneous technologies such as data mining, machine learning (ML), real-time analysis, various software platforms, operating systems, networking, and electronics for the efficient functioning of the system. The benefit of IoT is that the situation can be sensed and perceived as per the information which is gathered by devices on a real-time basis [1]. The term can be stated as the internet of medical things (IoMT), which includes sensors connected with mobile devices to gather data and further combined with electronic health care records.

As per data analytics companies, the market size of the IoT has reached $130B in 2018 and by 2023 it will touch $318B. According to IDC worldwide technology, spending on the IoT is likely to reach $1.2T in 2022. The global IoT market will grow from $157B in 2016 to $457B by 2020.

IoT is going high in and around all the fields whether it is engineering, business, or medical [2]. There are massive application areas and the one emerging area is health care and health monitoring as shown in Figure 1.1.

When IoT is applied for health care purposes, it combines the utility of the internet with apps and devices to deliver accurate real-time statistics of patients to the health providers to diagnose the information [3]. IoT in health management offers additional care for the patients outside the hospitals by doing monitoring of remote patients, sensing emergencies, and focusing on individual care [4].

There are various applications of IoT in health care such as telemedicine, BP monitors, clothes with a sensing device, pulse oximeters, glucose monitor, headset measuring brain waves, wearable devices to monitor heartbeats, devices to monitor sleep disorder, count walk steps, infant monitoring, and many more [5, 6].

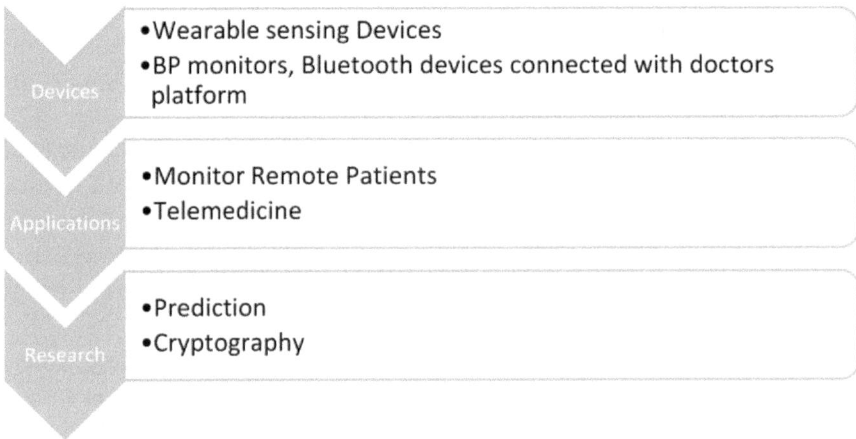

FIGURE 1.1 Applications and services of IoT in health care.

1.1.1 ADVANTAGES OF IOT IN HEALTH CARE

IoT is ruling health care in many positive prospects. It provides cheap and personal care to the patients [7, 8]:

1. **Cost-Effective:** As the IoT is providing real-time monitoring of patients, it will reduce the cost of lab checkups, doctor visits, and readmissions.
2. **Improved Disease Management:** Having the IoT supported health care devices, patients get a fast diagnosis of diseases with its accurate treatment and an emergency can be easily sensed.
3. **Individual Care:** Patients are more relaxed as they have a feel of individual attention since health care devices with IoT provide devoted care, better diagnosis of disease, and early processes treatment.
4. **Enhanced Outcomes of Treatment:** It permits the patients to stay home. The IoT supported devices of health care are empowered by sensors to gather data and to analyze it for further treatment. The collected data is transferred to doctors or hospitals so that patients can get enhanced treatments.
5. **Observing Remote Patients:** This is an actual benefit of tele-health, which can be achieved simply by smartphone. It will create an impression of home care to the patients who do not have good

facilities of hospitals and doctors in their locality. Patients can be monitored and inspected at their home and can be treated efficiently [9]. The elder people who are not able to approach hospitals are given personalized care at home.

6. **Maintenance of Real-Time Health care Record:** A centralized health care is delivered by IoT health care services, which in turn, also maintain the health care record in a well-organized manner. The data retained by monitoring devices can be sent to doctors, labs, or technicians for further diagnosis of diseases in the future as well.
7. **Improved Management of Health care Wastage:** Timely collection, prompt, and accurate display of patient information as well as its transference to the doctor leads to precise diagnosis and thereby leading to negligible chances of any health care wastage. Chances of unnecessary investigation or unduly delay are thereby reduced.
8. **Decline in Errors:** Clerical errors, printing mistakes, communication gaps, misinterpretation of values, or data are almost unknown due to the usage of smartphones and IoT thereby leading to a quantum reduction in error chances.

The technology for health care involving IoT is still developing. It is facing some challenges like security, data integration, privacy, etc. The rest of the chapter focuses on recent trends, infrastructure, application areas, and security issues related to IoT in health care.

1.2 RECENT TRENDS IN HEALTH CARE

Applying IoT in health care can be used to observe remote patients. Users can watch their fitness through apps, wearable devices, or sensing devices.

Apple watch series are newly launched to monitor fitness, heart rate, count calories, etc. Recently, people in Sweden installed a chip in their fingertips. The chip can share the data regarding the functioning of the body so that any flaws can be detected in an early stage. A trial has been done by using Bluetooth devices combined with a system tracking app that was experimented for cancer patients of neck and head by a group named CYCORE [10]. The device retrieves data of weight, blood pressure, symptoms, and responses to doctors and nurses regularly. A perceptible difference is noticed between the group of patients with a regular visit and the CYCORE group. The CYCORE received less severe symptoms and better treatment in comparison to other groups. Most recent smartphones are being launched with health sensors in the accessories like wrist gear.

A KHARE (Kinect HoloLens Assisted Rehabilitation Experience) platform is created by Microsoft Enterprise Services with INAIL (National Institute for Insurance against Accidents at Work) for mirror neuron therapy. Physicians are allowed to watch physical therapy sessions through the platform which allows real-time transmission of data [11].

Another example is Weka Smart Fridge which stands for storing information about vaccines. Remote monitoring can be done to confirm the vaccines are managed at the right temperature and proper storage place.

The analysis illustrates that when technology is combined with health care it improves patients' condition in a better way as they receives direct contact with doctors and facilities consistently to maintain good health. Currently, numerous examples exist show that the implementation of the IoT in the health care industry provides more vigilance towards health.

1.3 IOT INFRASTRUCTURE FOR HEALTH CARE AND HEALTH MONITORING

Abundant applications are brought by IoT in health care such as observing patients in remote areas and integrating with smart sensors and devices. Due to which patients are healthy and happy as they are getting care regularly without visiting hospitals [12, 13].

IoT infrastructure enables machine-to-machine interactions and data transfer on a real-time basis with medical devices [14]. Infrastructure includes various factors such as privacy of data, communication protocols, physical devices, cloud computing, security, and cryptography techniques used by experts for assessments and accurate automatic treatments. Communication also includes the concept of cloud computing [15].

IoT infrastructure consists of health care devices that sensed data further which is connected to a network as described in Figure 1.2. Health care devices may be hardware or software components. Sensors are capable enough to retrieve accurate data for further analysis. Connectivity may be done via wired or wireless connection [16]. Analysis of data can be based on a description of data or maybe by some calculations or maybe by some predictions. The data is further analyzed by their experts on their application platform such as their monitor device. Topology, architecture, and platform are the backbones of infrastructure: The topology includes physical configurations, activities, and communications. Architecture stands for the organization of software and hardware in the system including connection with other physical devices. Framework, library, and environment are part of the platform [17].

The associated technologies are big data, ML, mobile computing, cloud computing, IoT, cryptography, and cybersecurity. The data accumulated is so enormous that we need to include the technology of big data to manage it. All the apps functions and data transfer takes place through mobile without being connected by physical connection. Cloud computing plays a vital role to provide internet-based services very efficiently. All the devices whether wearable or non-wearable requires the IoT for connectivity and functioning.

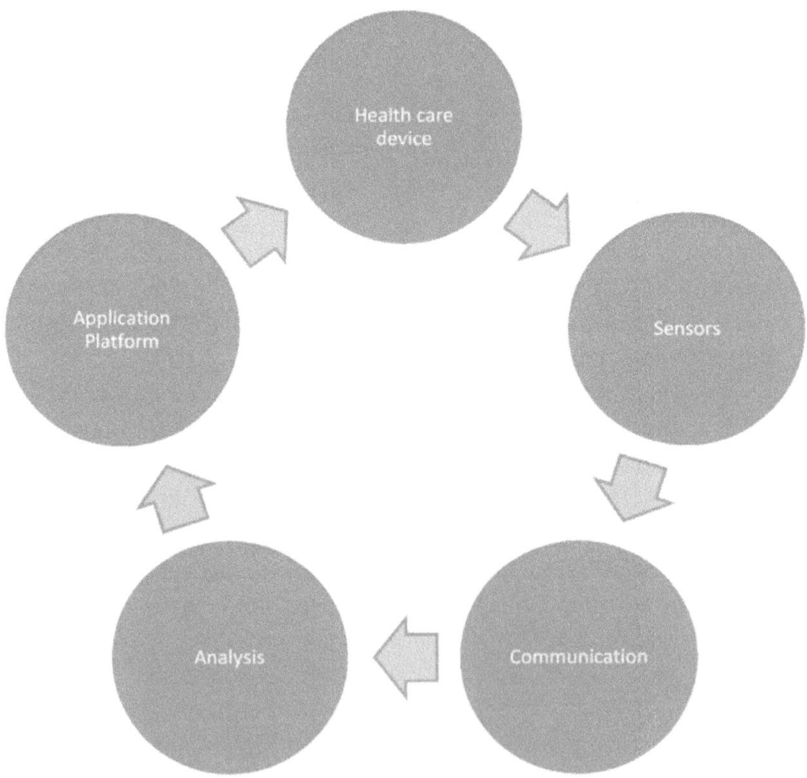

FIGURE 1.2 Conceptual architecture of IoT in health care.

Hackers and attackers are all around the world. The data collected belongs to patients and users are their general and sensitive information. As to keep data safe, cryptography has a major contribution. The system and data need to be secure from cyber-attack for which cyber laws are mandatory to implement.

The points to contemplate for infrastructure are selecting the right application platform for most of the values which can handle increased data load, can recover from failure, read accurate information from sensors, and communicate smoothly. It should be fast, accurate, and reliable so as it can be used effectively. Still, it has a lot of challenges regarding data security and the authenticity of users or experts.

1.4 APPLICATION AREAS

IoT health care devices have numerous benefits such as patient monitoring and communication, patient drug supply, electronic health implants, hospital and building management, patient engagement, and data collection [18, 19].

Nowadays, patients are getting faster health care [20]. Telemedicine is delivering health services and assistance in remote areas via communication technology.

1.4.1 TELEMEDICINE

From 1950, telemedicine is moving forward rapidly as it is playing a crucial role in the lives of people living in remote areas by solving the problems of people through video conferencing simply by smartphones or desktops. Doctors and patients can exchange information on different screens simultaneously. The patients not accessing medical facilities can connect the doctors on a live screen. Implementation of telemedicine is a beam of light for those developing countries which do not have good infrastructure, good technologies, and shortage of technical experts, lack of doctors, or physicians [21].

The definition of telemedicine given by WHO states that: *"The delivery of health care services, where distance is a critical factor, by all health care professionals using information and communication technologies for the exchange of valid information for the diagnosis, treatment, and prevention of disease and injuries, research, and evaluation, and for the continuing education of health care providers, all in the interests of advancing the health of individuals and their communities."—WHO* [22].

Telemedicine is offering great help to remote people in conjunction with IoT as shown in Figure 1.3. Telemedicine cannot be imagined without IoT. The infrastructure of IoT contributes to telemedicine as an audio-video transfer of data, exchanging of reports, and consultation without barrier.

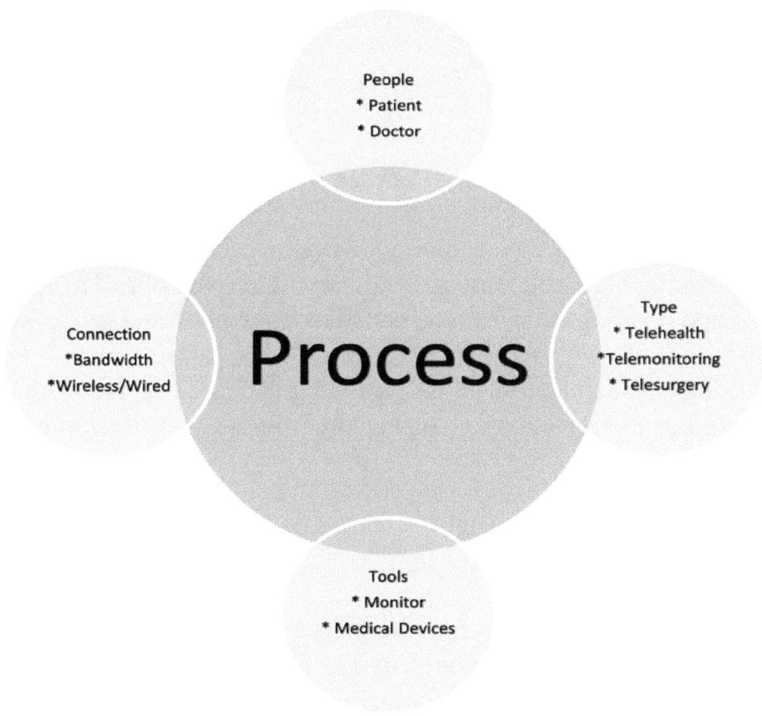
People
* Patient
* Doctor
Connection
*Bandwidth
*Wireless/Wired
Process
Type
* Telehealth
*Telemonitoring
* Telesurgery
Tools
* Monitor
* Medical Devices

FIGURE 1.3 Concept of telemedicine.

Many branches of medicine benefitting the users through telemedicine such as branch teleradiology is achieving good rates and providing good services.

The advantages of telemedicine are time-saving, cost-effective, privacy, no exposure to other communicable diseases through different patients, better follow up of patients, specialist consultation, and no geographic obstacle.

1.4.1.1 TYPES OF TELEMEDICINE SERVICES

1. **Telehealth:** Both the terms telemedicine and telehealth can be used interchangeably, even though there is a slight difference between them.

   Telehealth offers more scope of services in comparison to telemedicine such as training, medical education, administrative conferences, also non-clinical services additionally with clinical services like telemedicine.
2. **Telemonitoring:** The definition of telemonitoring suggested in the literature as the usage of information technology to observe the status of patient's health, while least concern about the geographic locations. The technology uses electronic devices with a combination of communication devices. Real-time health monitoring of patients decreases the gap between diagnosis and treatment.

   Telemonitoring permits patients to observe their health and fitness at home without doing a doctor's visit. The data is automatically collected by sensors and electronic equipments and transferred to the respective doctor. Usually, patients suffering from heart ailments and chronic asthma are benefitted by telemonitoring.
3. **Telesurgery:** It is a technique to perform surgery irrespective of distance with the help of robotics and technology. With the remarkable use of technology such as robotics, sensing devices in medical science operate patients on long distances. Remote surgery is a boom in medical science which eradicates geographic obstructions to provide timely and quality surgery.

1.4.2 CLOTHES WITH SENSING DEVICES

A lot of innovations in designing of clothes are equipped with sensing devices; for example, commuter jackets having sensing devices in sleeves to guide directions without reaching the phone. Newly designed socks are available which are capable to measure foot pressure. Smart shirts are designed respective to athletes for monitoring heart rate, stress level, and anaerobic threshold. Smart sleeves are created to monitor heart rate. Wearable electronics in clothes have key components in its architecture [23]:

1. **Power Providers:** To get energy for its smooth functioning.
2. **Sensors:** These are the crucial part of electronics designed for the clothes.
3. **Chip for Data Storage and Analyzing:** It is required for data processing.
4. **Communication:** Maintain connectivity between various components.

1.4.3 BP MONITORS

A wireless device that syncs with the health cloud displays a chart that can be visualized on the iPhone or any android phone to monitor blood pressure and heart rate. It is very easy to use with a reliable reading of measurements and provide instant feedbacks. Advantages of such BP monitors are:

1. Observing accurate blood pressure;
2. Automatic wireless sync with an app;
3. Understandable visualization charts;
4. Can have good connectivity both wired or Bluetooth;
5. Compatible with Android or iOS.

Many adults are affected by hypertension and cannot afford to go hospitals for medical checkups regularly. Such BP monitors offer precise information to them which in turn is a great help for them.

1.4.4 LIGHT WEIGHT HEALTH CARE DEVICES

1. **Pulse Oximeters:** It is a wireless device used to measure how much oxygen present in the blood. The painless device is attached to the finger to read blood flow, sense data, and display the reading. It sends beams of light for reading oxygen in the blood and to read pulse rate. The calculated outcome is displayed on the screen after processing the data. It can also be connected to the ear lobule. The benefits of the device are:
   - i. small and lightweight;
   - ii. reliable;
   - iii. durable; and
   - iv. battery indicator.

2. **Glucose Monitor:** It automatically measures the glucose level in the blood. It collects the data about glucose level and its rate of change. A real time-based glucose monitoring device make the patients feel stress-free throughout the day. It provides round the clock blood sugar variations assessment. Diabetic patients can have their blood sugar charting done for glucose monitoring.

   Better control by being prescribed medicines according to variations. Unconscious and comatose blood sugar assessment can do even remotely to avoid grave complications. Sometimes machines are inserted in the body part (e.g., in the arm) to monitor glucose level and transmit the data in every few minutes through wireless transmission.

The insulin pen is also beneficial to patients who depend on insulin. It measures the type, time, and amount of insulin in a given dose.

1.4.5 CARDIOVASCULAR DEVICES

Cardiovascular diseases are most dangerous all over the world; generally causing loss of life. Nowadays, the discovery of IoT supported cardiovascular devices reduce the risk of attack and make life better. Such devices can regulate heartbeat, detect the formation of blood clots, monitor calories consumed, observe physical activities, and can predict a heart attack. Some examples of such devices are mentioned as examples.

For rhythm control-pacemakers, biventricular pacemaker and implantable cardioverter defibrillator are used. Pacemakers and biventricular pacemakers are implanted under the skin of the chest, which passes the signals and controls the heartbeat to a normal rate. The data is collected by a doctor from the pacemaker for further analysis. Pacemaker helps many users to lead a normal life. A cardiac loop recorder is also an IoT health care device that records the heart rhythm. These devices are still the concern point for the researchers as they are too much prone to cyber-attacks. Holter monitor devices can be used for regular ECG monitoring in patients even at home.

Sudden abrupt changes in ECG in predisposed patients can be used to prevent arrhythmias and cardiac arrest.

1.4.6 WEARABLE DEVICES

Wearable devices are beneficial to maintain fitness as they provide time-to-time information regarding pulse rate, sugar level, and many more [24].

Intelligent asthma management is an empowered real-time respiratory monitoring system to maintain fitness. Smart contact lenses are used measure the glucose level in diabetic patients from their tears. Small watch-style devices are used to count walk steps, breathing rate, and heart rate to maintain fitness.

Health patch MD is an innovative technology including biosensors, ECG electrodes, and three-axis accelerometers to monitor heart rate, breathing, temperature, and position of a body in case of a fall.

Wearable asthma solution is a kind of wearable health care device which can diagnose an attack of asthma before it occurs so that patient can take immediate action.

Headset measuring brain waves is a wearable EEG meditation headset. A small headset that can be fit on the head includes sensors to measure activity. It reads the brainwaves and detects stress levels and oxygen levels in the brain. A smart posture corrector helps to improve the posture by vibrating as the posture goes wrong by tracking the posture. It introduces a healthy life while improving the posture during sitting and walking. It maintains the data on the Android or iOS app on monthly or weekly basis.

The major parts for the functioning of wearable devices are:

1. **Audio Component:** Actuators such as speakers make it happen.
2. **Sensor:** They collect information from either or both ambiance and user both.
3. **Power:** Requirement defines the type of power or its source needed.
4. **Data Storage:** Data is retrieved through sensors placed in wearable devices viz. wristwatch. Finally, the gathered data is stored in a computer or any smart devices for permanent storage.
5. **Microcontroller:** Small discrete comfortable microcontrollers are made for the ease of users; many of them are available in attractive colors and washable material.
6. **Communication:** Wireless connectivity needed for communication with devices via Wi-Fi, Bluetooth, etc.
7. **Display:** Actuators such as LEDs make it happen.
8. **Location Sensitizer:** Done by sensors, especially the location sensors (GPS).

1.5 SECURITY ISSUES

Manufacturers are providing various devices to customers rapidly. But we should ponder whether they are efficacious on security issues or not.

There may be numerous glitches in the security that may arise as a deficiency of visibility in key issues related to security. It may be hacking of IP address at home or office, which may be data leaked or other issues [25]. Health care devices are an interesting focus of hackers. It is one of the inimitable challenges for security in IoT health care devices [26].

Some security issues are discussed here, they may be:

1. **Unsuccessful Testing and Updating of IoT Health Care Devices:** Presently, there are billions of IoT health care devices used by people all over the world. Insufficient automatic updates are the prime security concern. The keenness of manufacturers to launch their products somewhere vanished the perception of security in their devices.
2. **Setting Default Passwords:** Those devices set with default passwords are very prone to cyber-attacks. Weak passwords can easily be hacked by attackers and data can be infected. So, it is been suggested that users should modify their credentials as soon as possible as they receive the health care device.
3. **Unrecognized Communication Protocols:** Some IoT health care devices use unknown protocols for communication which increases the probability of attack. Outdated infrastructure for communication is a big alarm for such IoT devices.
4. **Privacy and Security of Huge Amount of Data Generated:** Enormous amount of data is generated due to IoT health care devices for which privacy and security cannot be overlooked. The data when it is accessed, shared, processed, and analyzed by the different users need extra caution while transmission. It requires some legal and tough rules regarding privacy. Unused data should be removed very efficiently.
5. **Better Sensors:** There is still a huge gap in the availability and accuracy of available sensors for health care. It is a deep need for better sensors in the health care domain for better outcomes.

1.6 SECURITY METHODOLOGIES

As there are valuable benefits of IoT-enabled health care devices, security issues cannot be ignored [27]. There are several things to be defended against these attacks [28].

As the market of IoT health care devices is increasing rapidly, the risk of cyber-crime is also growing very fast. Manufacturers and health care industries must concern about the privacy and security of data related to patients. It must fulfill integrity, authenticity, and scalability issues of security as it deals with the private information of users:

1. **Applying Authentication on Various Factors:** There should be a multifactor authentication process to improve security. Authentication combined more than two factors which may include login credentials, date options, identification marks, OTP, fingerprints, etc. Usually, it improves security as it is difficult for hackers or attackers to retrieve and break all the authenticity factors. The multi-authentication factors can be divided into three parts:
    - Knowledge factor which includes login credentials;
    - Possession factor which includes OTP; and
    - Inherence factors such as biological traits, for example, fingerprints. Reliability increases as the security system include multifactor authentication.
2. **Encryption of Data:** As the health care devices are vulnerable to cyber-attacks, there should be key factors defined for privacy to keep the confidentiality of records. The data related to patients should be given to authorized experts. That data can be easily hacked while communicating through a network. Whether it may be general data which includes general information, or sensitive data which includes data regarding fertility status or infectious disease of patients, it makes to be sure that data should not be leaked to unauthorized users [29]. So, encryption techniques must be applied for improving trust and the relationship between user and company. Encryption techniques for IoT health care include Data Encryption Standard, Advanced Encryption Standard, RSA encryption, etc.
3. **Installation of Antiviruses or Intrusion Prevention Software:** Antivirus software or intrusion prevention software should be installed in health care devices involving desktop or smartphone. It will help and reduce the chance of an attack on the data.

4. **Automatic Security Updates:** The remarkable suggestion for reducing the risk of cyber-attacks is to upgrade health care devices automatically. The inability to upgrade automatically is the key challenge for the health care industry. The operating system, anti-viruses, and firmware required to be enhanced automatically.
5. **Recovery from Failures:** Technology should be advanced such as devices that can recover from failure without loss of information. Generally, equipments are connected to cloud computing, which improves the efficiency of the system to recovery from failure. There may be systematic markers or alarm clocks to alert the users to save data till checkpoints.

Abnormal conditions should be identified to reduce the risk of failure. A proper recovery plan must be designed before using IoT health care devices.

1.7 CHALLENGES

In medical science, IoT is used for improving the functioning of health care devices but it faces a lot of challenges which cannot be ignored:

1. **Data Management:** The data is collected on a large scale by health care devices whether from wearable devices or non-wearable devices. That data is heterogeneous and needs to be analyzed rapidly.
2. **Scalability:** In the health care industry, huge data is gathered and the system should be capable enough to manage it efficiently. The computing process is to be capable enough to use and investigate the data and should be adaptable to change.
3. **Interoperability:** Devices need to be more flexible to communicate. The equipment should be more powerful for exchanging information regardless of physical configuration and architecture.
4. **Outlier Analysis:** The major challenge to the health care industry is to identify the outlier values from the collected data. Many times, the data gathered may be erroneous, altered, and hacked. So, it is difficult to detect those values that are deviated from the data set.
5. **Design Issues:** It is tough to improve design issues as technology is growing very rapidly. It is because of a lack of good computing resources, deficiency of worthy sensing devices, and limited energy.

1.8 CONCLUSION AND FUTURE SCOPE

Getting care of health is the basic right of any civilian. Sometimes it is very costly and tiring to reach the hospital for regular checkups. Many areas in various countries do not have basic facilities for medical.

But stretching of IoT in health care is a very innovative concept as it delivers unparalleled benefits. Currently, IoT enacting a crucial role in health care and health monitoring. Technology is beneficial to patients for monitoring their health at home instead of going to hospitals daily. There is improved treatments, simultaneous reporting and monitoring, direct connectivity, and regular data analysis by physicians. IoT is altering the health care industry by innovative and beneficial devices and by providing monitoring of remote patients. IoT-enabled health care devices offers individual attention to patients.

IoT is still tackling challenges regarding security issues. IoT needs attention to security and applying encryption techniques while transmitting and receiving data at both ends. In the future, IoT in health care must include encryption of data for the protection of information. Manufacturers and providers of IoT health care devices must ensure data security to their users. In the future, health care needs to more efficient and intelligent to tackle the challenges with associating with new technologies such as artificial intelligence, big data, and ML.

The chapter presents the perception of the IoT in health care devices with its infrastructure and challenges. It can be concluded that the IoT is redefining health care and health monitoring.

KEYWORDS

- **cardiovascular devices**
- **challenges**
- **future scope**
- **internet of medical things**
- **internet of things**
- **security methodologies**
- **telemedicine**

REFERENCES

1. Dziak, D., Jachimczyk, B., & Kulesza, W. J., (2017). IoT-based information system for health care application: Design methodology approach. *Applied Sciences*. doi: 10.3390/app7060596.
2. Sethi, P., & Sarangi, S. R., (2017). Internet of things: Architectures, protocols, and applications. *Journal of Electrical and Computer Engineering.* Article ID 9324035. doi: https://doi.org/10.1155/2017/9324035.
3. Velasco, C. A., Mohamad, Y., & Ackermann, P., (2016). Architecture of a web of things e-health framework for the support of users with chronic diseases. *Proceedings of the 7th International Conference on Software Development and Technologies for Enhancing Accessibility and Fighting Info-Exclusion* (pp. 47–53). ACM. doi: 10.1145/3019943.3019951.
4. Bhunia, S. S., (2015). Adopting internet of things for provisioning health-care. *ACM International Joint Conference on Pervasive and Ubiquitous Computing.* ACM. doi: 10.1145/2800835.2801660.
5. Ma, X., Wang, Z., Zhou, S., Wen, H., & Zhang, Y., (2018). Intelligent health care systems assisted by data analytics and mobile computing. *Wireless Communications and Mobile Computing,* Article ID 3928080. doi: https://doi.org/10.1155/2018/3928080.
6. Aranki, D., Kurillo, G., Yan, P., Liebovitz, D. M., & Bajcsy, R., (2016). Real-time telemonitoring of patients with chronic heart failure using a smartphone. *IEEE Transactions on Affective Computing*, 206–219. doi: 10.1109/TAFFC.2016.2554118.
7. Jita, H., & Pieterse, V., (2018). A framework to apply the internet of things for medical care in a home environment. *Proceedings of the 2018 International Conference on Cloud Computing and Internet of Things* (pp. 45–54). ACM. doi: 10.1145/ 3291064.3291065.
8. Hu, F., Xie, D., & Shen, S., (2013). On the application of the internet of things in the field of medical and health care. *IEEE International Conference on Green Computing and Communications and IEEE Internet of Things and IEEE Cyber, Physical, and Social Computing.* IEEE. doi: 10.1109/GreenCom-iThings-CPSCom.2013.384.
9. Babu, B. S. K., Srikanth, T. R., & Narayana, L., (2014). IoT for health care. *International Journal of Science and Research (IJSR)*, 322–326.
10. Kevin, P., et al., (2011). Cyberinfrastructure for comparative effectiveness research (CYCORE): Improving data from cancer clinical trials. *Translational Behavioral Medicine*, 83–88. doi: 10.1007/s13142-010-0005-z.
11. Kent, C., (n.d.). *Health care*. Retrieved from: https://www.medicaldevice-network.com: https://www.medicaldevice-network.com/comment/bringing-internet-things-healthcare/ (accessed on 29 July 2020).
12. Purri, S., & Kashyap, N., (2018). Augmenting health care system using internet of things. *8th International Conference on Cloud Computing, Data Science and Engineering (Confluence).* Noida, India: IEEE. doi: 10.1109/CONFLUENCE.2018.8443002.
13. Mishra, P. A., & Roy, B., (2017). A framework for health-care applications using internet of things. *International Conference on Computing, Communication, and Automation (ICCCA).* Greater Noida, India: IEEE. doi: 10.1109/CCAA.2017.8230001.
14. Bui, N., & Zorzi, M., (2011). Health care applications: A solution based on the internet of things. *Proceedings of the 4th International Symposium on Applied Sciences in Biomedical and Communication Technologies.* ACM. doi: 10.1145/2093698.2093829.

15. Renta, P. T., Sotiriadis, S., & Petrakis, E. G., (2017). Health care sensor data management on the cloud. *Proceedings of the 2017 Workshop on Adaptive Resource Management and Scheduling for Cloud Computing.* ACM. doi: 10.1145/3110355.3110359.
16. Khalil, N., Abid, M., Benhaddou, D., & Gerndt, (2014). Wireless sensors networks for internet of things. *IEEE 9th International Conference on Intelligent Sensors, Sensor Networks and Information Processing (ISSNIP)* (pp. 1–6). IEEE.
17. Islam, S. M., Kwak, D., Kabir, M. H., Hossain, M., & Kwak, K. S., (2015). The internet of things for health care: A comprehensive survey. *IEEE Access, 3*, 678–708. doi: 10.1109/ACCESS.2015.2437951.
18. Khan, R., Khan, S. U., Zaheer, R., & Khan, S., (2012). Future internet: The internet of things architecture, possible applications, and key challenges. *Proceedings of the 2012 10th International Conference on Frontiers of Information Technology* (pp. 257–260). doi: 10.1109/FIT.2012.53.
19. Farahani, B., Barzegari, M., & Aliee, F. S., (2019). Towards collaborative machine learning driven health care internet of things. *Proceedings of the International Conference on Omni-Layer Intelligent Systems* (pp. 134–140). ACM. doi: 10.1145/3312614.3312644.
20. Mora, H., Gil, D., Terol, R. M., Azorín, J., & Szymanski, J., (2017). An IoT-based computational framework for health care monitoring in mobile environments. *Sensors*. doi: 10.3390/s17102302.
21. WHO, (2010). *Telemedicine Opportunities and Developments in Member States.* WHO.
22. WHO Group Consultation on Health Telematics (1997: Geneva, Switzerland). (1998). *A Health Telematics Policy in Support of WHO's Health-for-all strategy for global health development: report of the WHO Group Consultation on Health Telematics,* 11–16 December, Geneva, 1997. World Health Organization. https://apps.who.int/iris/handle/10665/63857.
23. Kaur, K., (2012). *Azosensors.* Retrieved from www.azosensors.com/article.aspx?ArticleID=84: https://www.azosensors.com/article.aspx?ArticleID=84 (accessed on 29 July 2020).
24. Metcalf, D., Milliard, S. T., Gomez, M., & Schwartz, M., (2016). Wearable's and the internet of things for health: Wearable, interconnected devices promise more efficient and comprehensive health care. *IEEE Pulse, 7*(5), 35–39. doi: 10.1109/MPUL.2016.2592260.
25. Tarouco, L. M., Bertholdo, L. M., Granville, L. Z., & Arbiza, L. M., (2012). Internet of things in health care: Interoperability and security issues. *IEEE International Conference on Communications.* IEEE. doi: 10.1109/ICC.2012.6364830.
26. Sicari, S., Rizzardi, A., Grieco, L., & Porisini, A. C., (2015). Security, privacy, and trust in the internet of things. *Computer Networks: The International Journal of Computer and Telecommunications Networking, 76*, 146–164. doi: 10.1016/j.comnet.2014.11.008.
27. Roman, R., Najera, P., & Lopez, J., (2011). Securing the internet of things. *Computer, 44*(9). doi: 10.1109/MC.2011.291.
28. Baker, S., Xiang, W., & Atkinson, I. M., (2017). Internet of things for smart health care: Technologies, challenges, and opportunities. *IEEE Access*. doi: 10.1109/ACCESS.2017.2775180.
29. Sun, W., Cai, Z., Li, Y., Liu, F., Fang, S., & Wang, G., (2018). Security and privacy in the medical internet of things: A review. *Security and Communication Networks*. doi: https://doi.org/10.1155/2018/5978636.

CHAPTER 2

Antennas for Biomedical Applications

SHAILESH and GARIMA SRIVASTAVA

Ambedkar Institute of Advanced Communication Technologies and Research, Delhi–110031, India,
E-mail: shailesh.jayant404@gmail.com (Shailesh)

ABSTRACT

This chapter presents the possibility of implantable biomedical devices (IMD) in the ongoing years. Various people all over the world are presently relying upon implantable devices to improve their health. An implantable antenna for biomedical applications is a key part of a transmitter. Implantable biomedical antennas are widely utilized and most fitting as an alternative to the intricate medical services. Implantable biomedical antennas are utilized for the people and as well as for the animals. The implantable biomedical antennas are utilized for constant checking of body temperature and blood pressure, tracking the dependent individuals or lost pets, and exchanging health records remotely from the implanted antenna in the human body, for example, pacemaker to an outside radio frequency receiver. As such, watching patients distantly can be recognized without having any direct physical contact. Biomedical telecommunication allows the exchange of information from "on-body to off-body," or from "on-body to on-body," or from "in body to off-body." The motivations behind implantable biomedical antennas are remote health checking, ailment treatment, stomach-related observing, hyperthermia, and finding the area of the tumor. The difficulties looked by utilizing these implantable antennas comprises of the design and implantation of these antennas in the human body because the human body is lossy. While structuring the implantable antenna, the accompanying parameters should be viewed as like conservative size, significantly less weight, safety, and successful work inside the medical frequency band (industrial, scientific, and medical

(ISM) radio bands, medical implant communication services (MICS), and so on), wide working bandwidth and high radiation efficiency for ease and comfort of the patients. The main theme of this chapter is to present the design and difficulties of different sorts of implanted antennas. Additionally, simulation and measurement methods and results of implanted antennas are studied. Moreover, this chapter gives an overview of biocompatibility and safety issues.

2.1 INTRODUCTION

Since numerous people around the world are suffering from many severe diseases and having critical health conditions, many researchers are interested in implantable biomedical devices for exploring solutions for different drastic medical conditions. These implantable devices are installed under the skin or on the body surface of the patients to examine the physiological signals of the human body. These physiological signals are transmitted to doctors through wireless communication. This is one of the main advantages of the biomedical implantable device since the patient need not go to the hospital for the daily checkup and the condition of the patient's health is analyzed wirelessly by the doctor. Another advantage of the biomedical device is the tracking of humans and pets such as dogs and cats, which can be done easily with the help of these devices. The main section of the implantable devices is the antenna through which the signal is sent or transmitted. Therefore, the excellent design of these types of an antenna is very crucial. Since the implantable devices are to be installed inside the human body, the size and the weight of the antenna should be less.

The wireless implantable system is very useful in biomedical telemetry and the implantable biomedical antenna is a very important part of the wireless implantable system [1, 2]. The wireless communication uses implantable antennas for the real-time monitoring of the patient's body temperature, pH, and glucose. For the ease and comfort of patients, the antenna's size and weight should be less. But this results in poor gain and efficiency.

Another issue with the implantable antennas is the high power dissipation in tissue nearby the implantable biomedical antenna. The maximum transmitting power is determined such that the specific absorption rate (SAR) regulation limits are not violated. ANSI/IEEE rules for peak SAR averaged over 1 g of tissue is 1.6 W/Kg. Like mobile phones, implantable biomedical antennas should have SAR less than or equal to 1.6 W/Kg over

1 g of tissue, so that the less electromagnetic (EM) energy is absorbed by the body; otherwise, this may harm the patient rather than providing cure from disease.

A wireless implantable system which has the application of biomedical telemetry consists of a sensor, implantable antenna, power supply, and insulation. The main motive of this system is the transmission of information from the human body to an external base station. Therefore, the transducer provides physiological signals and transmits these signals by using the operator through an implantable antenna [3]. Before designing the biomedical antenna, the surrounding environment circumstances must be considered. These circumstances are represented by the circular stratum demonstrating working habitat as shown in Figure 2.1. The first stratum contains origin which denotes air. The second one denotes biocompatible padding. The third and fourth stratum denotes the human tissue layer.

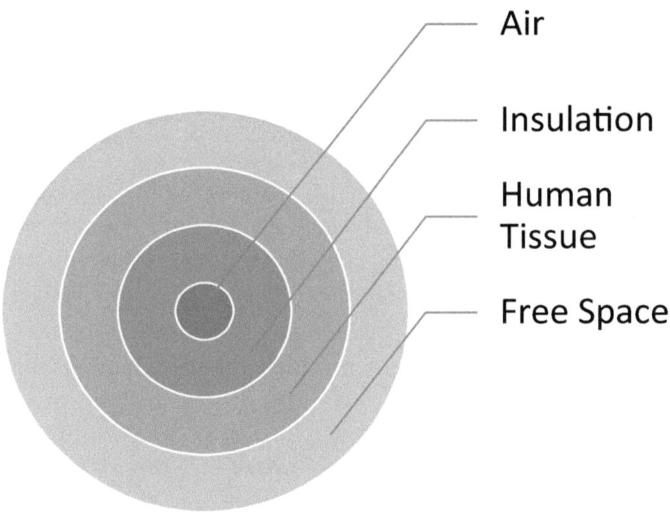

FIGURE 2.1 Body sample: muscle, skin and fat [3].

2.2 TYPES OF IMPLANTABLE ANTENNAS

So far, various types of implantable antennas have been proposed for biomedical applications, and some of them are categorized in Figure 2.2. These antennas are categorized as a slot antenna, dipole antenna, antenna array, circularly polarized (CP) antenna, and other kinds of antennas.

2.2.1 SLOT ANTENNAS

The slot antenna contains slots of different shapes and sizes such as circular, rectangular, etc. These slots are etched out from the metal. These slots radiate EM waves as same as a dipole antenna. These antennas are used in ultra-high frequencies (UHF) and microwave frequencies. The two types of slot antennas such as open-ended slot feed antenna and slot antenna with meandered slot are explained in the further sections.

2.2.2 DIPOLE ANTENNAS

The dipole antenna mainly contains two conductors having equal lengths and a feed line connected between them. The dipole antenna can also be used in radar applications. The three types of dipole antennas such as dipole antenna with meandered line structure, folded dipole antenna, and on-chip implantable dipole antenna are explained in the further sections.

2.2.3 ANTENNA ARRAYS

The antenna array is the combination of various antenna elements that work as a single antenna. This improves the gain and directivity of the antenna. The antenna array is used in designing MIMO (multiple input multiple output) antennae, which enhances the signal reliability. The two types of antenna arrays such as LCP substrate-based antenna array and textile array with textile EBG (electron band-gap)-based antenna are explained in the further sections.

2.2.4 CIRCULARLY POLARIZED (CP) ANTENNAS

The CP antenna is a type of antenna having circular polarization. This antenna reduces the multipath interferences from the reflected signals. Thus, this type of antenna is used in many applications such as satellite communication, direct broadcasting services (DBS), wireless local area network (WLAN), Worldwide Interoperability for Microwave Access (WiMAX), wireless personal area networks (WPAN), etc. The five types of CP antennas such as capacitively-loaded CP antenna, CP loop antenna, ground radiation CP antenna, broadband CP antenna, and a CP antenna with wide axial ratio (AR) are explained in the further sections.

2.2.5 OTHER ANTENNAS

The five different types of antennas for biomedical applications in this section such as stacked PIFA (planar inverted F antenna), zeroth-order resonance antenna, flexible antenna, dual-mode (heating/radiometry) antenna, and differentially fed dual-band antenna are explained in the further sections.

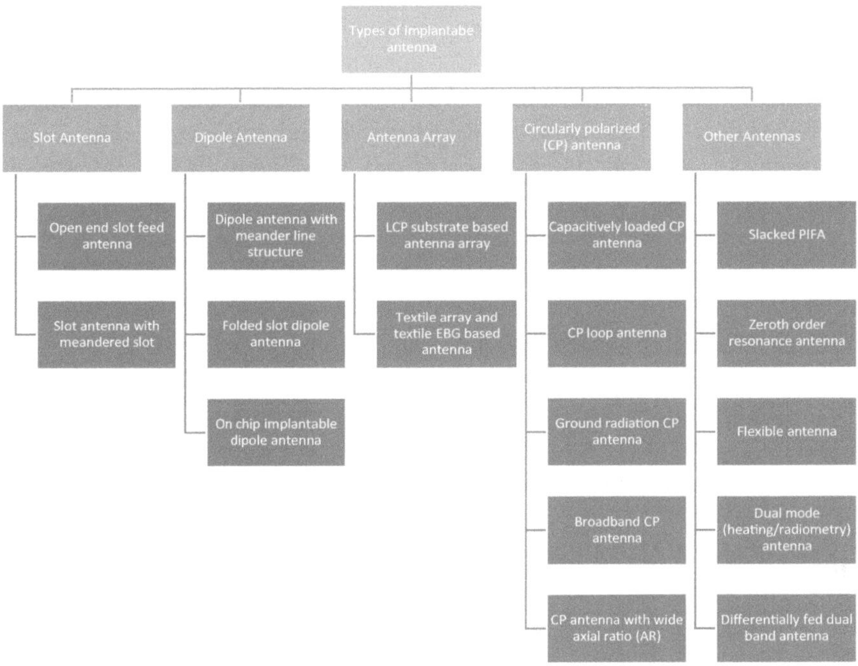

FIGURE 2.2 Types of implantable antenna.

2.3 SLOT ANTENNA

In this section, we will discuss slot antenna with open-end feed and meandered slot.

2.3.1 OPEN-END SLOT FEED ANTENNA [4]

This type of antenna is used in the biomedical telemetry for transmitting the physiological signals from one location to another location. There are three sorts of a biomedical implantable antenna in WBAN application, such as on-body antenna, off-body antenna, and in body antenna. In on-body antenna, information can be exchanged in both off-body and in body antenna and uses the surface of the human body as a transmission medium for the EM waves. The on-body antenna is used in real-time monitoring. When an antenna is placed on the human body, the antenna has a high SAR, conservative structure, and moderate reflection coefficient. There are different types of challenges faced in the design of the on-body antenna like the performance of the antenna must not affect the human body and the radiation must be adjusted to minimize the hyperlink loss.

The patch's length, width, and ground are calculated with the design equations (1 to 6), which are shown in Ref. [4]. The open-end slot feed is utilized for decreasing different microstrip losses. The inherent matching of the antenna impedance is accomplished by presenting open-end space. The open-end slot feed line improves the antenna's gain and bandwidth. To increase the current conveying path, the antenna's patch has two arms and each arm is partitioned into two sections. A compact ground structure is utilized for reducing the return loss. To lessen the mutual coupling effect with different antennas, a defected ground structure (DGS) is utilized. Figure 2.3(a) shows the transmitting patch and Figure 2.3(b) shows the structure of the ground of this antenna.

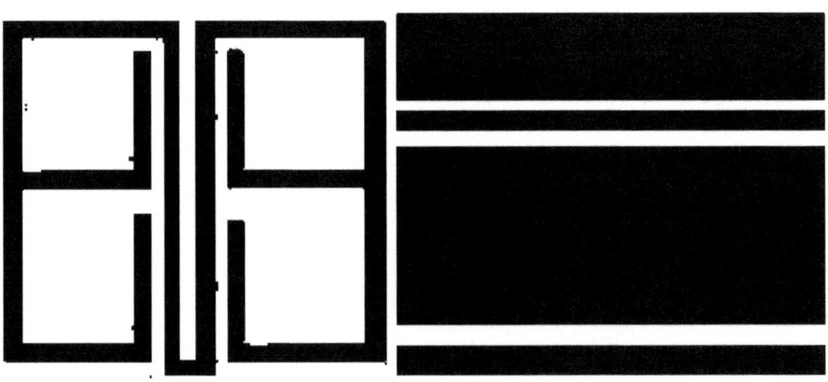

(a) (b)

FIGURE 2.3 (a) Structure of top layer, (b) Structure of bottom layer [4]

The phantom model is shown in Figure 2.4. The antenna is located at a distance of 10 mm from the phantom model.

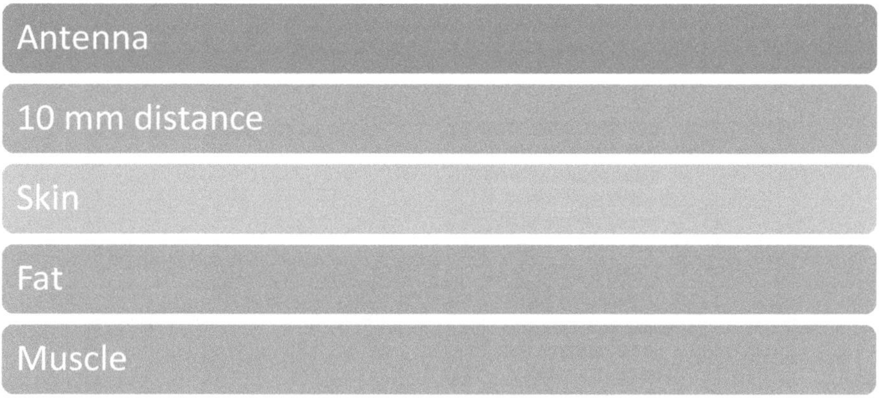

FIGURE 2.4 Human Phantom Model [4]

2.3.1.1 ADVANTAGES

- This type of antenna is compact and flexible.
- It improves the bandwidth and reflection coefficient.

2.3.1.2 APPLICATIONS

- It enhances the signal to noise ratio for the microwave imaging system.
- It can be used to detect various kinds of cancer.
- It is used for on-body communication and in the biomedical sector because of its SAR = 0.039 W/Kg.

2.3.2 SLOT ANTENNA WITH MEANDERED SLOT [5]

There are numerous types of antennas like microstrip antenna; PIFA, meandered dipole, and slot antenna are introduced for miniaturization of the antenna. Furthermore, human bodies are lossy and affect the antenna performances. The insulating layers are used to decrease power loss and rise the antenna's gain. Insulations can provide power enhancement. Additionally, by considering that no magnetic losses in the human tissues, magnetic supply decrease power that is absorbed as compared to the electric one of the same model. Therefore, the design of the magnetic field slot antenna is chosen. Figure 2.5 presents the structure of this antenna, which is operating at the MICS band. The detailed parameters are given in Ref. [5].

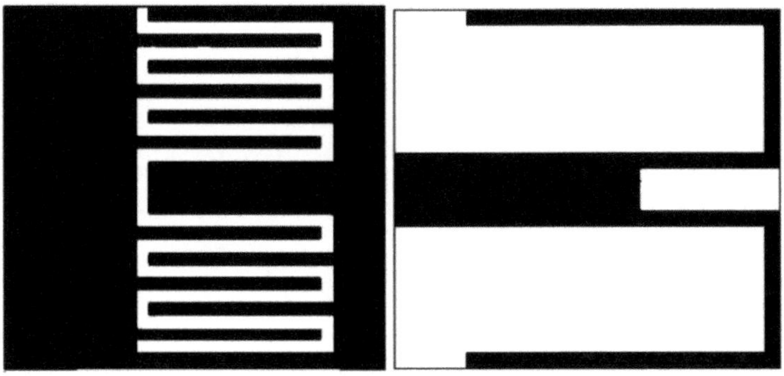

(a) (b)

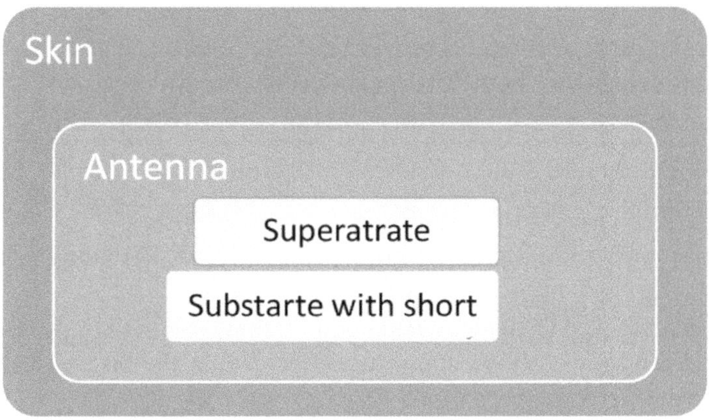

(c)

FIGURE 2.5 Slot antenna with meandered line (a) Top View, (b) Bottom View, (c) Side view of antenna implanted into skin model [5].

The antenna's performance is measured using a plastic container that is filled with skin-mimicking gel to confirm the simulation results. The CST Gustav human voxel model is used to test the robustness of the antenna, which represents a male having a weight of 69 kg and a height of 176 cm. This antenna is implanted into the arm. The results of both slot antennas are presented in Table 2.1.

TABLE 2.1 Slot Antennas

Antenna Type	Open-End Slot Feed Patch Antenna [4]	Open-End Slot Antenna [5]
Year	2019	2013
Band	ISM	MICS
Volume (mm^3)	2030	139.7
fo (GHz)	2.45	0.402
BW (%/GHz)	16%/0.39	28.3%/0.115
Gain (dBi)	7.2	–27.7
SAR 1 g W/Kg	0.039	<1.6
PT (mW)	1	3.9
Substrate	Teflon	Rogers
Dielectric constant	2.1	10.2
Return loss (dB)	–46.64	>–10
Simulation tool	CST	CST
Model	Three-layer human phantom model	One layer skin model and arm of human model/human voxel model of the arm
In Vitro	nd	Skin mimicking gel

Note: nd = not defined, BW = bandwidth, PT = input power allowed.

2.4 DIPOLE ANTENNA

In this section, we will discuss the dipole antenna with a meander line structure, folded slot, and on-chip implantable antenna.

2.4.1 DIPOLE ANTENNA WITH MEANDER LINE STRUCTURE [2]

The implanted antennas need to be designed with less chip area and weight for patient's relief and ease of implantation process. But, miniaturization ruins the gain and the efficiency of the antenna. The antennas such as planar inverted-F antennas (PIFA), dipole antennas, and the loop antennas are introduced to provide miniaturization. The planar folded dipole antenna has a compactness of 20 mm^3 and a good gain of –27 dB. These parameters are better than other types of antennas. Moreover, another difficulty in the design of implantable antennas is high power dissipation in tissues near the antenna except for high gain and compactness.

The resonance frequency of this antenna depends on the total trace length. The dipole antenna's trace length is around 27 mm for each arm at 402 MHz. So as to shorten the dipole, the meandering line section in each arm of the antenna is used. As presented in Figure 2.6, the proposed meandering section replaces a certain part of each arm. This design increases trace length with no increase in the dimensions of the antenna.

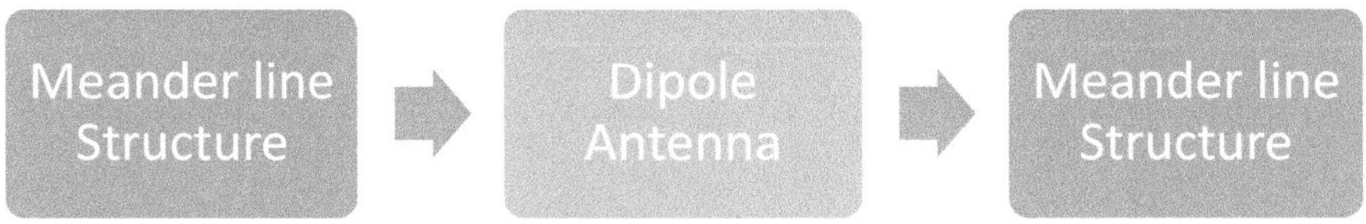

FIGURE 2.6 Dipole antenna with meander line structure [2].

With the purpose of increasing gain and efficiency, the meander line arrangement at the ending of each dipole arm is placed. So as to confirm the significance of the straight-line section (W1), efficiency is determined as a function of W1/W2. With the use of thin substrate/superstrate layers, further miniaturization can be achieved.

A cylindrical three-layer model, which is similar to the structure to the human arm, is shown in Figure 2.7. This antenna is located inside the dermis (underneath the skin surface).

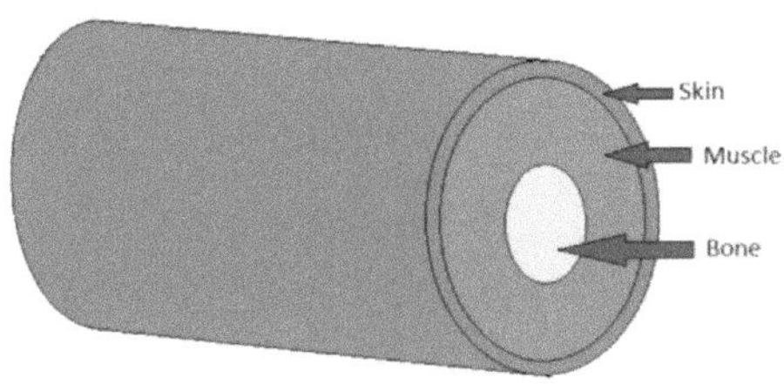

FIGURE 2.7 Cylindrical shaped three layer model [2].

2.4.2 FOLDED SLOT DIPOLE ANTENNA [6]

This antenna is like a flexible folded slot dipole, which is embedded in the biocompatible PDMS, because folded slot dipole has the ability to deliver wide bandwidth as compared to patch antennas. The top and the front view of the antenna are presented in Figures 2.8 and 2.9, respectively. The structure of the folded slot dipole antenna is shown in Ref. [6]. The folded slot dipole antenna has an operating frequency of 2.45 GHz in the ISM band. The superstrate along with the substrate of PDMS are used in the design. A single layer of liquid which is mimicking human muscle tissue is added below the substrate and on top of the superstrate. Flexible electronic technology is used to manufacture the antenna. A coplanar waveguide (CPW) having 50 Ω impedance is used as the feed for a slot dipole antenna.

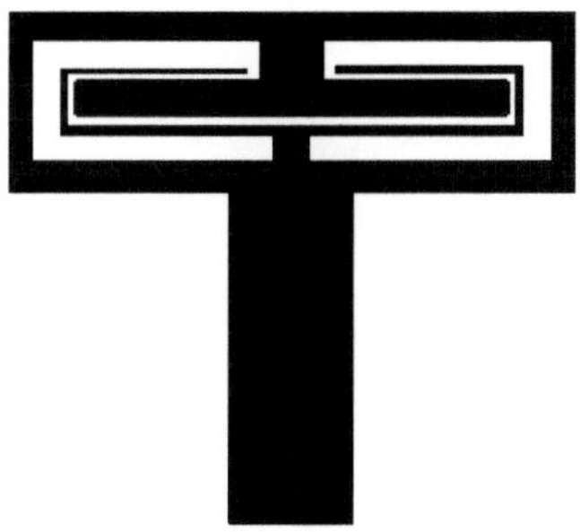

FIGURE 2.8 Coplanar waveguide-fed antenna (Top View) [6].

2.4.3 ON-CHIP IMPLANTABLE DIPOLE ANTENNA [1]

The implantable antennas like PIFA, slot antenna (H-shaped cavity), loop antenna, a dipole antenna, CP patch antenna, etc., are not small enough to be implanted in heads, eyes, organs, or blood vessels, etc. To address this issue, CMOS technology is used to further decrease the size of less than 1 cubic millimeter of the antenna and to achieve the integration of the antenna and radio frequency (RF) circuits on a single chip. This antenna contains differential-feeding which acts as an output balun for making an integrated system efficient and compact. The CMOS technology not only reduces the cost but also improves the power efficiency of the transmitter and receiver noise performance. The antenna structure contains two spiral lines connected as arms of the dipole antenna as shown in Figure 2.10(a). The current vectors in the spiral wire can be arranged such that the resonance frequency is lowered for the given length and size of the spiral wire, when current vectors are always in reinforcing directions of the indirectly adjacent wires. For simulation, ground-signal-ground-signal-ground (GSGSG) pads are added. The dipole antenna's resonance frequency is determined by the current vector alignment of each arm and capacitive coupling between arms and feeding locations.

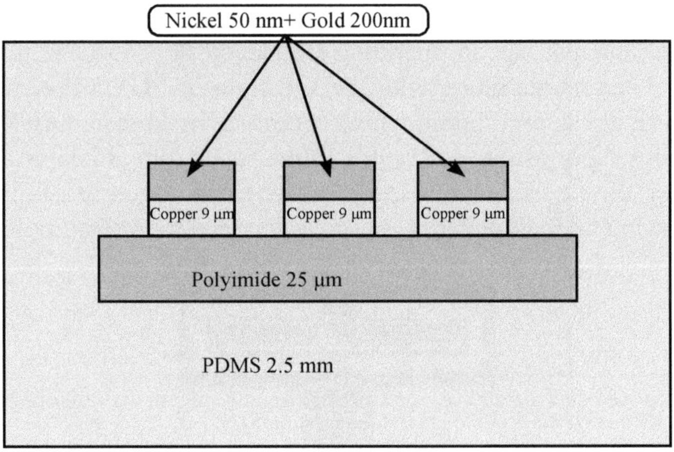

FIGURE 2.9 Coplanar waveguide-fed antenna (Front View) [6].

A dipole antenna is located at a distance (*d*) from top of the skin tissue as presented in Figure 2.10(b). This antenna has a wide impedance bandwidth (0.7–1.1 GHz). But, the exterior dipole antenna has a small shift in resonant frequency with the variation in the distance (*d*). The antenna is implanted inside the human head of the Gustav voxel human body. Additionally, the proposed antenna's impedance matching in the human head is much improved than that in the skin phantom. The coupling strength is around –56 dB at 902 MHz, which is similar to the value of ~–58 dB in the skin phantom at the same frequency. This antenna is embedded in the skin phantom for validating the design. The results of dipole antennas are presented in Table 2.2.

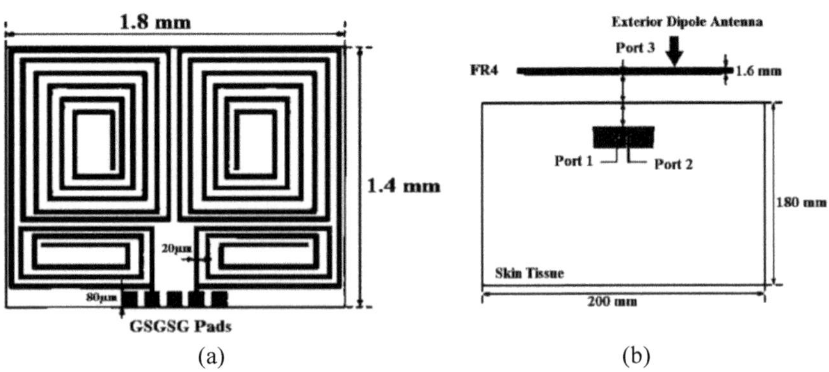

FIGURE 2.10 (a) Structure of on-chip antenna; (b) Simulation setup [1].

TABLE 2.2 Dipole Antennas

Antenna Type	Dipole Antenna (Meander Line) [2]	Folded Slot Dipole Antenna [6]	Dipole Antenna with CMOS Technology [1]
Year	2018	2011	2016
Band	MedRadio	ISM	ISM
Volume (mm3)	20	22.5	0.77616
fo (GHz)	0.402	2.45	0.915
BW(%/GHz)	35%/0.1396	0.0835	0.4
Gain (dBi)	–23.7	–23.98	Nd
SAR 1 g W/Kg	<1.6	0.308/10 g	134.15
PT (mW)	5.9	2	11.9
Substrate	Rogers	PDMS	Rogers
Dielectric Constant	10.2	2.2	10.2
Return Loss (dB)	–27	–20	<–10
Simulation Tool	nd	ADS/CST	CST
Model	Cylindrical three-layer model	Human model arm	Single-layer skin model, Voxel Gaustav human head model
In Vitro	Gel and Liquid	Liquid	Nd

Note: nd = not defined, BW = bandwidth, PT = input power allowed.

2.5 ANTENNA ARRAY

In this section, we will discuss antenna arrays based on the LCP substrate and textile array.

2.5.1 ANTENNA ARRAY WITH LIQUID CRYSTALLINE POLYMER (LCP) SUBSTRATE [7]

Recently, the terahertz frequency band has various applications in medical diagnostics due to its small form factor, broad spectral bandwidth, high spectral resolution, and so on. But, antennas with high gain are needed for better reception and transmission and as well as for terahertz signal, since at terahertz frequencies, the path loss is very high. As the patch loss is reasonably low at a number of transmission windows across the spectrum of terahertz frequency, terahertz transmission can be accomplished at these low loss frequencies to enhance wireless link reliability. In contrast with other types of antennas having THz applications, microstrip-based patch antenna can fulfill the stated necessities—such as manufacturing—of terahertz antenna and is challenging due to short wavelength at THz frequencies. The incorporation of the antenna with other terahertz components is crucial for getting compactness.

This type of microstrip patch antenna arrays (Figure 2.11) based on LCP substrate material contains five components, which are made at 0.835 THz, 0.635 THz, and 0.1 THz. The LCP-based material improves electrical performance in contrast with RT/Duroid material and has a thin substrate which can be intended to use in microstrip patch antenna with negligible surface wave effect. The design equations regarding this THz array are given in Ref. [8].

- **Advantage:** Improved gain with fabrication tolerance.
- **Application:** Vital sign monitoring and cancer detection (Skin and Liver) through THz spectroscopy.
- **Future scope:** More arrays with high gain can be made by stacking more numbers of this antenna parallel topology with feeding and by using impedance matching using rectangular waveguide (hollow).
- **Disadvantage:** SAR is not calculated for patient safety.

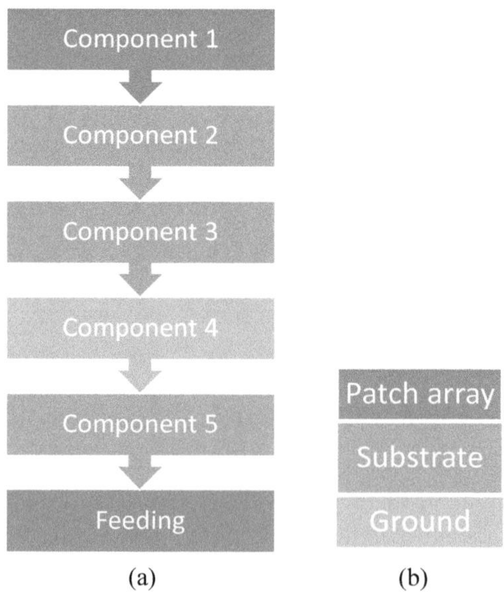

FIGURE 2.11 Geometry of the LCP substrate-based array; (a) front view (b) side view [7].

2.5.2 TEXTILE ARRAY AND TEXTILE ELECTROMAGNETIC (EM) BAND-GAP (EBG)-BASED ANTENNA [9, 10]

Wearable health monitoring systems are realized for biomedical applications such as Smart Shirt, VTAM Project, LifeShirt, European Wearable Healthcare System, etc. [10]. Such wearable clothing having various sensors can be made using textile materials and as well as it finds applications in electrocardiography, shock/fall sensors, respiration activities, and temperature. The wearable health monitoring can transmit information to the health personnel using mobile communication, WLAN, Bluetooth, etc. This is a cheap, flexible, and smart wearable textile array scheme. The word "smart" signifies to signal processing ability to combine antenna signals with different phases and amplitudes for determining the direction of arrival (DoA) of the transmitting sensor and consequently adjust the radiation pattern towards it.

For implementing DoA estimation and beamforming on curved human body parts like a human arm or head, two antennas with circular polarization are created using flexible materials. The gathered RF signals are then directed to super-heterodyne receivers, designed and fabricated in-house. Prior to a final amplification, bandpass filters filter these signals at both RF and IF frequencies, before and after frequency down-conversion to IF. Using the analog-to-digital converter, the afterward amplified signal is filtered again. This subsystem is presented in Figure 2.12.

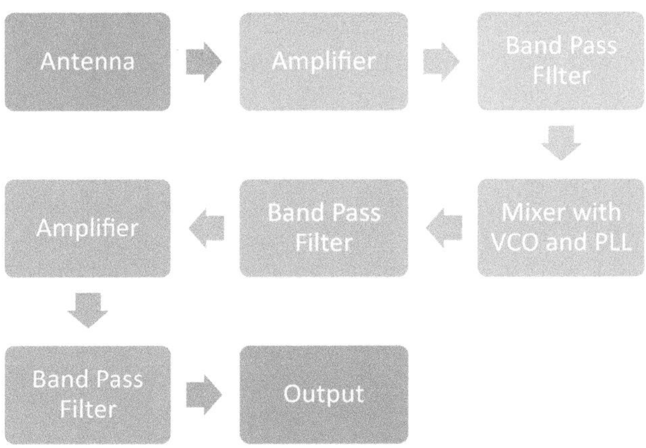

FIGURE 2.12 Block diagram of the receiver subsystem [10].

Circular polarization is created and used by a diagonal fed probe and chamfered edges, positioned diagonally at the opposite ending of a patch as shown in Figure 2.13. To make it suitable for application on different human body parts (e.g., male arm), the element spacing greater than $\frac{\lambda}{2}$ is preferred.

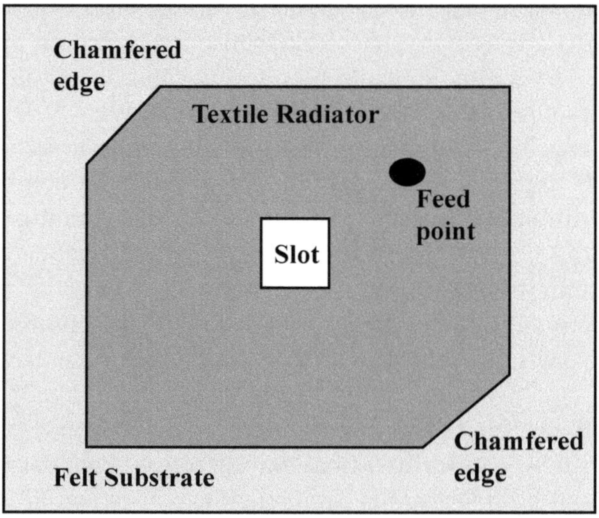

FIGURE 2.13 Fabricated prototype of single-element textile antenna fabricated prototype [10].

The curved human body phantom can be represented using two cylinders through different diameters (Figure 2.14). The antennas are placed on the cylinders which are filled with body emulating liquid.

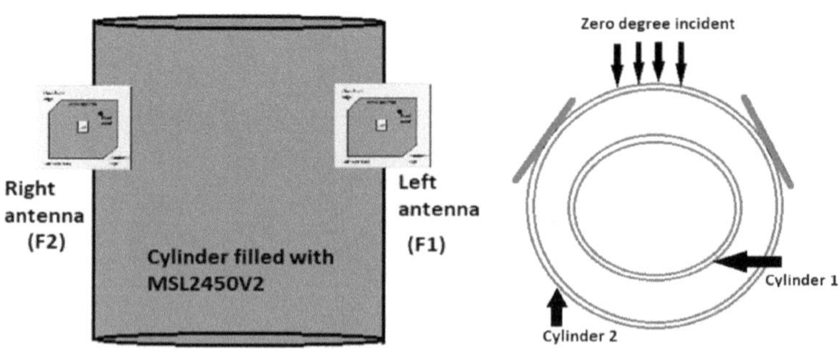

FIGURE 2.14 Two antennas are placed on cylindrical phantom [10].

Wearable computing systems have various applications in health monitoring, physical training, tracking, and emergency rescue [9]. Several designs of wearable antennas have a narrow bandwidth and a high front-to-back ratio. For providing less mutual coupling isolation from the human body and reducing SAR value, EBG structures are presented in wearable antenna. But, EBG structures suffer from an electrically large size antenna and poor front-to-back ratio. Wearable textile antennas combined with EBG structures can further decrease the antenna size without degrading the antenna's performance. EBG structure can generate phase reflection and suppress surface wave which results in a reduction in SAR and improvement in front-to-back ratio and gain; consequently, it increases the bandwidth of the antenna.

The inverse E-shaped monopole textile antenna is shown in Figure 2.15. A patch of the square loop having four T-shaped strip patterns is selected with the purpose of achieving a compact EBG structure. The strip pattern refers to the inductance. An EBG array is positioned on denim material. When the EBG reflection phase varies, it acts as an artificial magnetic conductor and when EBG suppresses the surface wave, it acts as a bandgap.

The antenna is positioned over the EBG structure as shown in Figure 2.16, so that to avoid short circuits, mismatch, and electrical contacts. Rohacell foam can be used as a spacer between the antenna and EBG. Rohacell foam is an extremely flexible foam which has the ability to take shape of nearby materials.

- **Advantage:** Enhances measured working bandwidth.
- **Disadvantage:** When the EBG is added, a little shift in resonant frequency is observed, which in turn creates a discrepancy in the fabrication and tolerance.

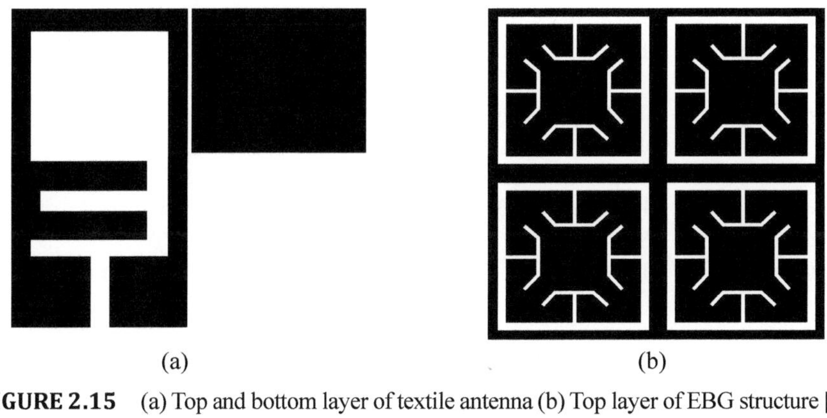

(a) (b)

FIGURE 2.15 (a) Top and bottom layer of textile antenna (b) Top layer of EBG structure [9].

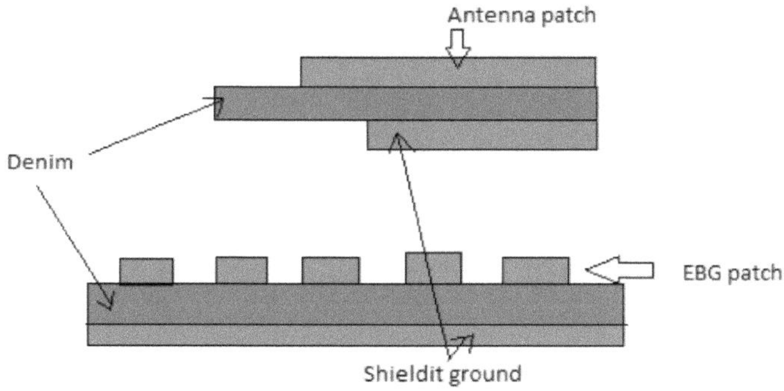

FIGURE 2.16 Antenna with EBG structure [9].

The results of antenna arrays are summarized in Table 2.3.

2.6 CIRCULARLY POLARIZED (CP) ANTENNA

In this section, we will discuss implantable antennas based on circular polarization such as capacitively-loaded CP antenna, CP loop antenna, ground radiation CP antenna, broadband CP antenna, and CP antenna with wide AR.

TABLE 2.3 Antenna Arrays

Antenna Type	Microstrip Antenna Array [7]	Smart Wearable Textile Array System [10]	Textile Antenna [9]
Year	2016	2013	2017
Band	nd	ISM	ISM
Volume (mm^3)	nd	nd	5078.4
fo (GHz)	0.835 0.635 0.1	2.39	2.4
BW (%/GHz)	24.3 17.3 1.8	0.312	27%/0.66
Gain (dBi)	16.37 16.52 15.82	4.9 dB	7.8 dB
SAR 1 g W/Kg	nd	0.014/10 g	0.0368
PT (mW)	1	nd	10
Substrate	Liquid crystal polymer substrate	Felt	Denim
Dielectric constant	2.91	1.45	1.7
Return loss (dB)	–30 –40 –38	–38	–45
Simulation tool	CST	CST	CST
Model	nd	Cylinder filled with body emulating liquid	Four-layer model
In vitro	nd	nd	nd
In vivo	nd	nd	Arm of a male volunteer

Note: nd = not defined, BW = bandwidth, PT = input power allowed.

2.6.1 CAPACITIVELY LOADED CP ANTENNA [11]

Due to multipath distortion, Communications through far-field RF linked telemetry can be hindered. CP radiation pattern is desirable in wireless access applications. Instead of using linear polarization, circular polarization can provide a decrease of multipath and as well as enhancement of bit rate errors. The capacitive loading gives better capacitive coupling and impedance matching for size reduction. The capacitively-loaded CP antenna is shown in Figure 2.17.

This antenna is placed inside the Gustav voxel human body. The resonant frequency is shifted because implant depth affects the resonant frequency and asymmetry of the human body affects polarization. To evaluate the effect of implant positions, single layer skin phantom and two cases of three-layer geometry (Figure 2.18) are simulated, wherein case one there is no gap between the antenna and fat layer, and in the second case, the antenna is positioned at some distance from fat layer. Based on the simulated results, the resonant frequency has some shift to a higher frequency when the antenna is inserted in the fat layer.

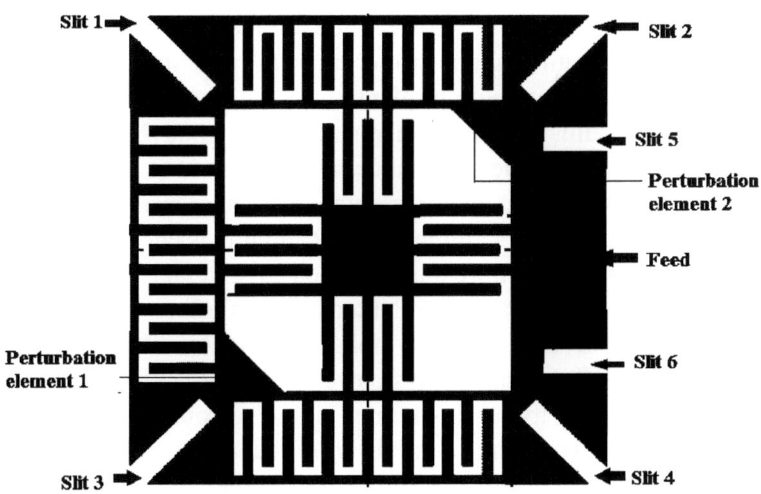

FIGURE 2.17 Geometry of CP implantable antenna [11].

- **Disadvantage:** Not covering the whole ISM band.

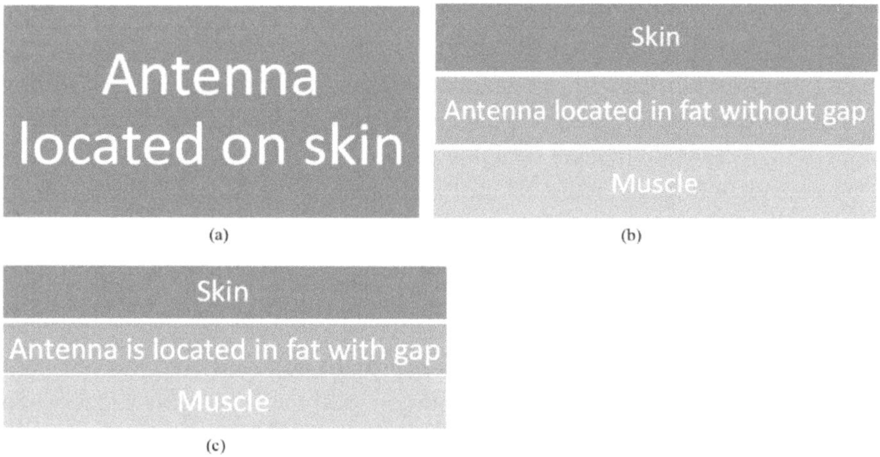

FIGURE 2.18 (a) single layer skin phantom (b) three layer tissue phantom (case1) and (c) three layer tissue phantom (case 2) [11].

2.6.2 CP LOOP ANTENNA [12]

It is problematic to find the correct location of the placement of the implanted system with respect to the external base station. Then again, the movement of patients with implanted systems supposed to be ensured under certain circumstances. As a result, for a good link between the implant system and exterior appliance, a CP antenna is desirable. These antennas are not dependent on the orientation of the transmitter and as well as the receiver. Generally, a single feed CP antenna is chosen, thanks to its trimness, in contrast with more than one feed CP antennas. The CP antenna in the base station as well as in implanted antenna offers an increase in the 3 dB gain as compared to a linearly polarized implantable antenna.

The broadband implantable system can deliver a high data rate and has superior tolerance to various human tissue surroundings. This system is necessary for the support of neural signal recording, cochlear implants, and high-resolution imaging. This CP loop antenna at the ISM band is introduced to enhance AR and bandwidth.

The design of the CP loop antenna is presented in Figure 2.19. This antenna contains a loop of square shape which is having a connection with four *LC* loadings. Four patches are connected to the loop at different quadrants with four high impedance lines independently. Moreover, the two shorting pins are located at I and III quadrants. This antenna is fed at quadrant IV and it is designed for right-hand circular polarization (RHCP). But, if the location of shorts and feed are mirrored along the x-axis, then left-hand circular polarization (LHCP) can be realized.

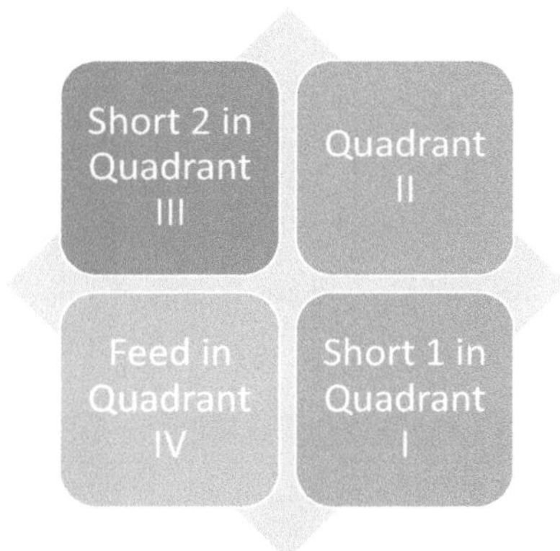

FIGURE 2.19 Structure of the CP loop antenna [12].

To validate antenna performance, antenna measurement is done in a plastic container, which is filled with pork and skin mimicking gel.

2.6.3 GROUND RADIATION CP ANTENNA [13]

With the intention of reducing the losses of multipath effect and achieving improvement in bit rate errors, less number of CP antenna is introduced. The two orthogonal field components (unaffected by transmitter or receiver orientations) can be excited by CP antennas with equal amplitudes and 90° phase difference. In Ref. [11], to operate at the ISM band, a capacitively-loaded CP antenna was introduced. But, it is sensitive to the change in environment and has a narrow AR bandwidth. The antenna design for the ingestible application of the CP helical antenna was also presented. This is a high profile helical antenna because of its multi-layer structure. Consequently, ground radiation implantable CP antenna was introduced and shown in Figure 2.21 and its simulation setup is shown in Figure 2.20. It has features such as low profile and wider AR bandwidth. This antenna finds the application in reliable communication and flexible implantation.

- **Advantages:**
  - Low profile design.
  - Wide AR bandwidth can be able to deliver decent robustness with the purpose of the good performance of antenna with different situations.

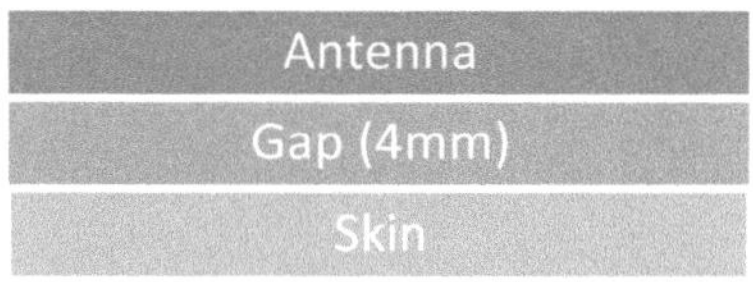

FIGURE 2.20 Antenna with a one-layer tissue phantom simulation setup [13].

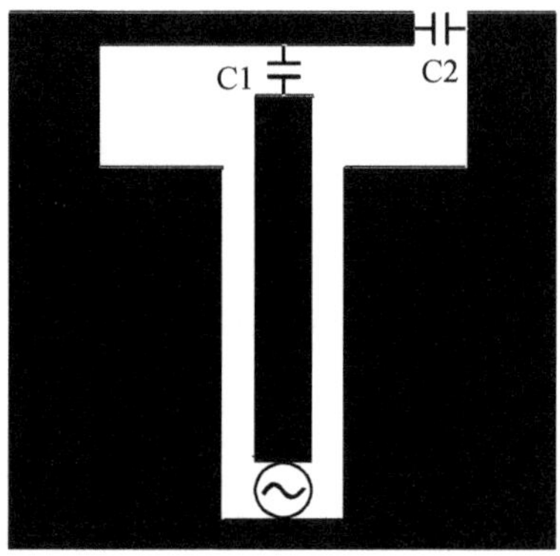

FIGURE 2.21 Ground radiation CP implantable antenna (top and side view) [13].

2.6.4 BROADBAND CP ANTENNA [14]

To decrease the effect of a shift in resonance frequency, the implantable antenna should be broadband. But, the electrically small size of implantable antenna results in a narrow bandwidth. Therefore, for wide bandwidth, some techniques have been used such as PIFA structure and stacked multilayer or CPW feeding antenna. Though, in stacked structure, fabricating and tuning operations are complex and in CPW feeding antenna, the backward direction is very strong to cause harm to the human body. Additionally, all the above-stated antennas are linearly polarized. In implantable antenna, because of different body postures and indoor multipath distortion, mismatch in polarization occurs, which results in bad communication quality. Because of this reason, circular polarization has been used. Circular polarization does not depend on orientation between receiver and transmitter and provides lower bit rate error, better mobility, and enhancement of stability of the link. The capacitively-loaded CP implantable antenna [11] is not able to cover the whole ISM band. Therefore, to address this issue of not covering the complete ISM band, broadband CP antenna is introduced. This antenna is designed using one layer planar structure. This implantable antenna has corner truncated and modified square ring microstrip antenna. So, to further increase impedance and AR bandwidth, a cross-shape slot is embedded in the ground plane with proper dimensions. Because of the wide impedance and AR bandwidth, this antenna is able to cover the complete desired band.

The geometry of this antenna is presented in Figure 2.22 and it is manufactured in Rogers's 3010 substrates and superstrate. The radiator on the top side of the substrate is modified as a square ring in place of the square patch because the current path is excited in the square ring than in the square patch for longer fundamental mode surface.

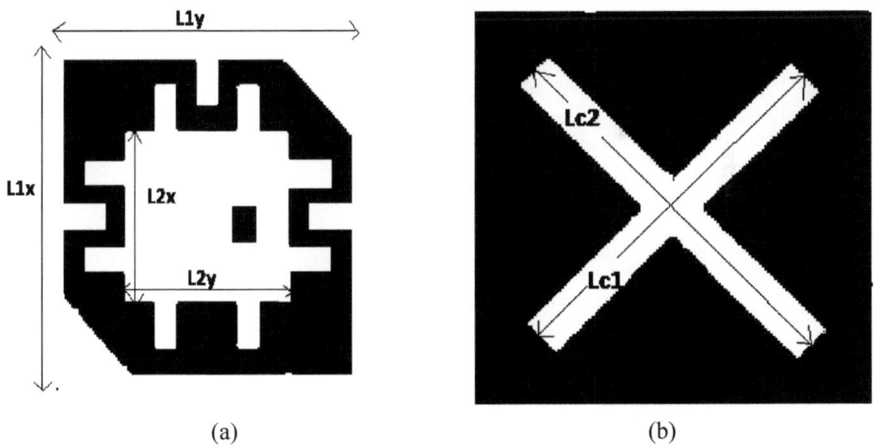

FIGURE 2.22 Broadband CP antenna (a) Top plane (b) Ground plane [14].

A human muscle tissue phantom in the HFSS simulator is shown in Figure 2.23. The antenna is positioned 5 mm away from the top of the cubic box. And this antenna is implanted into the left chest muscle of the CST Gustav voxel model to evaluate the effects of the human body on antenna performance. A plastic vessel filled with muscle mimicking liquid is used to validate the antenna performance. The recipe for muscle-mimicking liquid is given in Ref. [14].

2.6.5 CP ANTENNA WITH WIDE AXIAL RATIO (AR) [15]

The wide AR is an important characteristic of the implantable antenna because it provides decent tolerance to the human tissue and also provides high data exchange. So, this type of antenna has wide AR with a single-layered patch antenna because a single-layered patch antenna provides simple geometry, compact size, and good stability, but a multilayered antenna is a high profile antenna. The antenna structure as shown in Figure 2.24 has a center square slot with four slits, where these four slits are placed in parallel to each side of the patch. Also, two out of the four slits cut patch at the end. Additionally, at the diagonal of the center square slot, a pair of perturbation elements is presented.

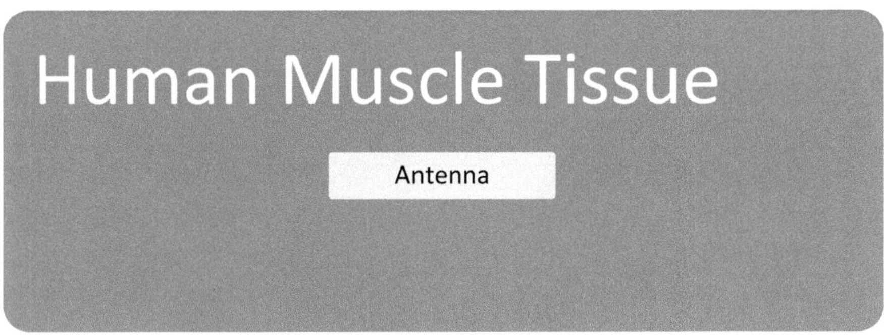

FIGURE 2.23 One layer tissue model [14].

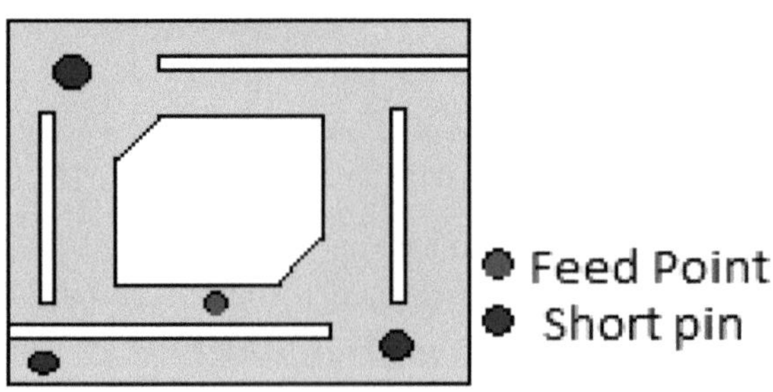

FIGURE 2.24 CP antenna with a wide axial ratio [15].

To estimate the sensitivity, this antenna is embedded in three different body phantoms, which are cubic single layer skin model, single layer scalp phantom, cylinder muscle phantom, and three-layer phantom (Figure 2.25).

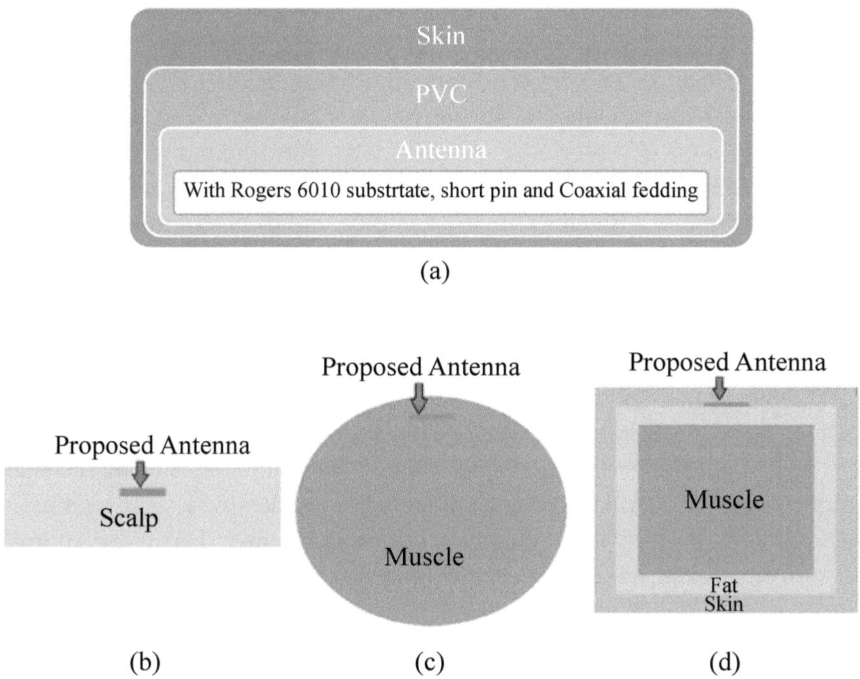

FIGURE 2.25 Various body models: (a) cubic single layer skin model (b) single layerscalp model (c) cylinder muscle model (d) threelayer phantom [15].

For measurement, minced pork and skin mimicking gel are used as human skin tissue models. The results of all CP antennas are summarized in Table 2.4.

2.7 OTHER ANTENNAS

In this section, we will discuss different types of implantable antennas based on different techniques such as stacked PIFA.

2.7.1 SLACKED PLANAR INVERTED F ANTENNA (PIFA)

The PIFA is used in wireless telemetry due to its flexibility in design and conformability [8]. The PIFA antenna is made from a monopole antenna. By the means of folding down the monopole to reduce the antenna's height and maintain identical resonating length, inverted L is created. The inverted L antenna looks like an inverted F antenna when feeding is applied to the inverted L. To obtain the PIFA, the planar element is used in place of the thin top wire of inverted F. Additionally, introducing a shorting pin between the ground and patch plane, increases the antenna's effective size. Therefore, there is a further reduction in physical dimensions [16].

In Ref. [8], skin implantable miniature PIFA in the Medical Implant Communication Service band is presented for biotelemetry. The testing of this antenna is done inside the skin tissue model, where the antenna is immersed by 2 cm inside a semi-filled plastic glass. The performance of the antenna is then examined inside the anatomical head model.

The stacked antenna (Figure 2.26) has a circular shape as the antenna is to be installed inside the anatomical head. This antenna is designed with a circular ground surface and dual meandered patches which are vertically stacked. Glue layers bond the dielectric layers together. The layers of high permittivity substrate are isolated by low permittivity glue layers, which results in a decrease in effective dielectric constant and electrical length of the antenna with an increase in resonance frequency. Meanders are equidistant by 1 mm and their width is small so as to increase the radiation area of the patch. A shorting pin is used for further miniaturization. For the detailed dimension of the stacked antenna, see Ref. [8].

2.7.2 ZEROTH ORDER RESONANCE (ZOR) ANTENNA [17]

The compact and broadband antennas are used to obtain size reduction and better performance for the biomedical applications. The antennas are suffered from the resonance frequency shift because of the change in the permittivity of the human body. The zeroth-order resonance antennas are introduced for MICS applications. To cover MICS bandwidth with 10 dB return loss and extremely compact size is obtained by the phenomenon of the epsilon negative zeroth-order resonance (ZOR). Additionally, the return loss of the antenna does not depend on the change in the electrical properties of the human body. This antenna (Figure 2.27) consists of a

TABLE 2.4 Circularly Polarized Antennas

Antenna Type	Capacitively Loaded CP Antenna [11]	CP Loop Antenna [12]	CP Ground Radiation Antenna [13]	Broadband CP Antenna [14]	CP Patch Antenna [15]
Year	2014	2013	2015	2016	2017
Band	ISM	ISM	ISM	ISM	ISM
Volume (mm^3)	127	214.6	54.95	127	127
fo (GHz)	2.455	0.915	2.45	2.45	2.4
BW (%/GHz)	7.7%/0.19	18.2%/0.161	18.2%/0.621	16.15%/0.39	6.2%/ 0.15
Gain (dBi)	–22	–32	–19.8	–17.16	–27.2
SAR 1 g W/Kg	213	599	356.4	254.74	nd
PT (mW)	7.51	2.6	<4.49	6.28	nd
Substrate	Rogers	Rogers	Taconic substrate	Rogers	Rogers
Dielectric Constant	10.2	10.2	2.95	10.2	10.2
Return Loss (dB)	<–10	<–10	<–10	>–10	>–10
Simulation Tool	HFSS/CST	HFSS	HFSS/CST	CST/HFSS	
Model	HFSS(Cubic skin phantom), CST (3D Gaussian Voxel Human Body)	Single layer skin model	Single and multi-layer tissue model	Gaussian Voxel model, HFSS Cubic box of human muscle tissue	Cubic one layered skin model
In Vitro	One layer skin material (solution)	Pork and Gel	Solid phantom	Muscle Mimicking Liquid	Gel and Pork
In Vivo	nd	nd	nd	nd	nd
AR				AR< = 3dB, 6.09%	

Note: nd = not defined, BW = bandwidth, PT = input power allowed.

radiating patch with CPW feeding and a bottom patch for decreasing the effect of the human body on antenna performance. Shunt inductance (L_L) is made by using two series chip inductors to obtain negative epsilon ZOR, which are attached between patch and ground plane. ZOR frequency is given by equation number (2.1):

$$\omega_o = \frac{1}{2\pi\sqrt{2C_R \times L_L / 2}} = \frac{1}{2\pi\sqrt{C_R \times L_L}} \tag{2.1}$$

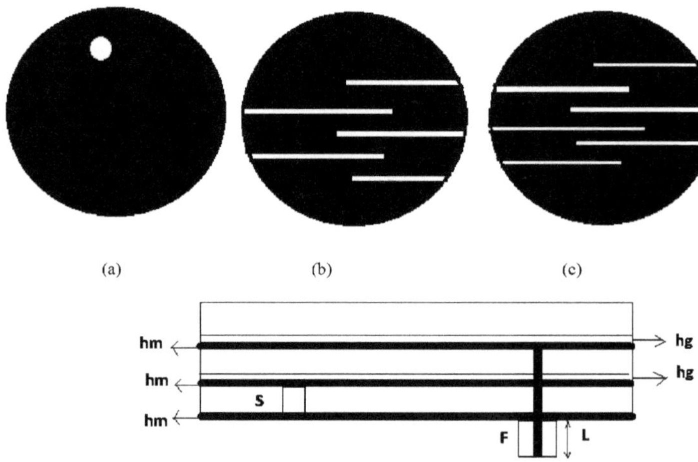

FIGURE 2.26 Slacked planar inverted-F antenna: (a) ground plane, (b) lower patch, (c) upper patch, and (d) side plane [8].

To verify the antenna's performance, the antenna is enclosed by a polycarbonate case and placed inside the human liquid phantom. The radiation pattern is dipole like in the air. But, in human liquid phantom, the radiation pattern is monopole like due to the conductive loss of the body. The low gain of –38dB is due to the high dielectric loss of the FR4 substrate.

2.7.3 FLEXIBLE ANTENNA [18]

In the field of biomedical telemetry, the different types of biomedical antennas are introduced. The previously introduced biomedical antennas do not have very good return loss, and no simulation or measurement test was done for the calculation of Sarthe cross-sectional view (see Figure 2.28).

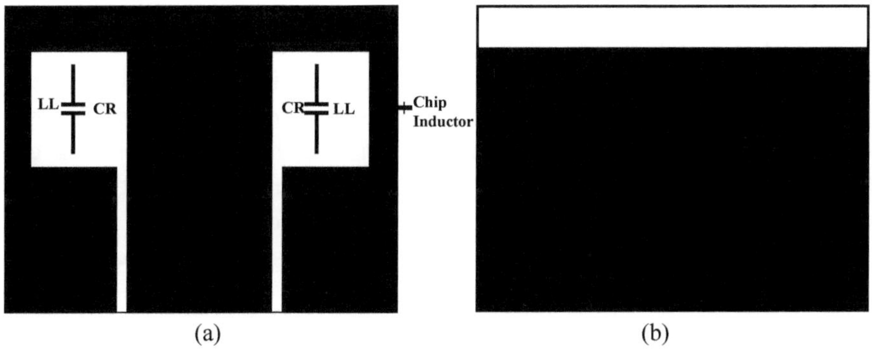

FIGURE 2.27 Structure of ZOR antenna (a) Top View (b) Bottom View [17].

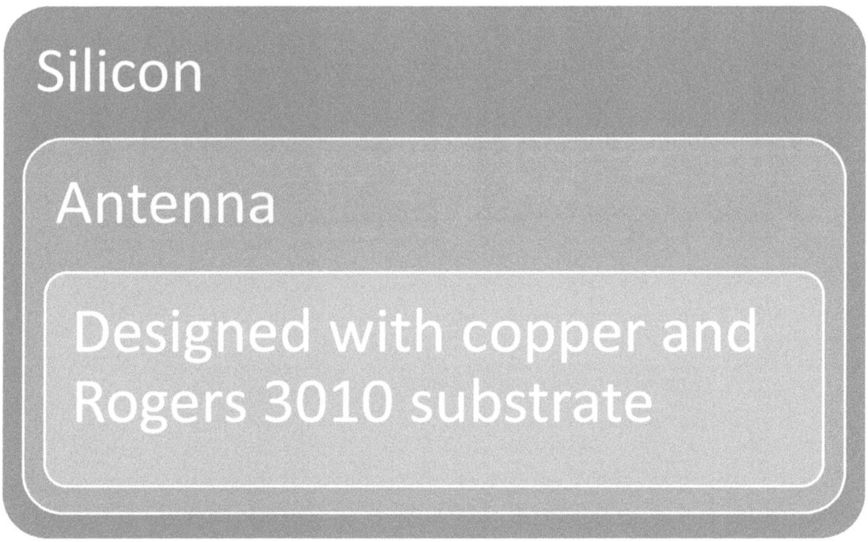

FIGURE 2.28 Cross-sectional view of flexible antenna [18].

The design of the antenna is presented in Figure 2.29. Antenna design is optimized by using cutting slots, where current distribution is very low. This process is repeated for various arrangements to get minimum return loss. The detailed list of optimized size parameters can be seen in Ref. [18].

The three-layer geometry model shown in Figure 2.30 consists layer of muscle tissue, fat tissue, and skin tissue.

The radiation pattern of this antenna is directional (prominent single-peak radiation). The antenna has high directivity focused at a direction, so that antenna would radiate away from the body except radiating into the body.

With the purpose of minimizing the discomfort of having an antenna inside the body, the antenna is designed to be thin in order that it can have flexibility with the body. Under distortion, resonant frequency shifts towards lower frequency. More shifts are observed in resonant frequency with higher bending of the antenna. The return loss also increases with the increase in the bending.

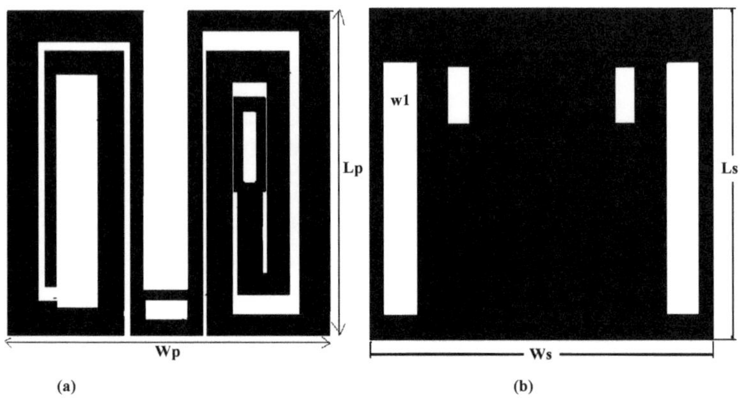

FIGURE 2.29 Antenna dimension (a) Patch (b) Ground plane [18].

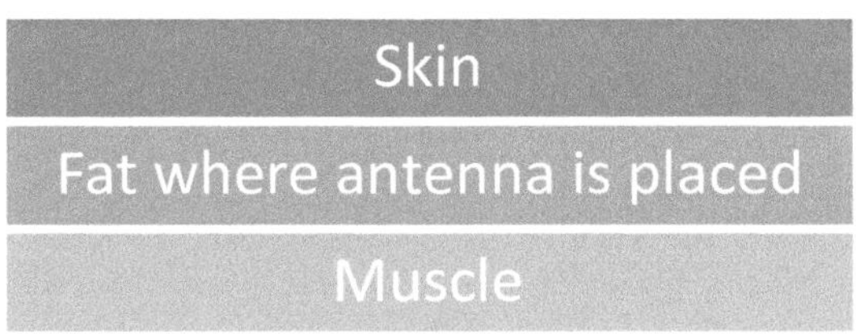

FIGURE 2.30 Antenna inside a three-layer skin model [18].

2.7.4 DUAL-MODE (HEATING/RADIOMETRY) ANTENNA [19]

In medicine, microwave heating and radiometry uses radio waves. Microwave heating is used for the treatment of hyperthermia of tumors and benign prostatic hypertrophy. In contrast, microwave radiometry is used for monitoring temperature during the treatment of hyperthermia.

Both microwave heating and radiometry can be used for monitoring tissue temperature in skin diseases and non-invasive medical treatment. For estimation of blood perfusion, tissue was primarily heated by the antenna and with the termination of the heating, radiometry read the rate of temperature decay.

The earlier dual-mode antenna containing annular slot antennas (ASA) and outer ASA are used for heating at 0.9 GHz, and a sinner one ASA is used for radiometry at L band. Though, the main challenges to overcome are in and out of band radio frequency interference (RFI). Therefore, this antenna introduces dual-mode RFI enhancement for heating (0.9 GHz) and radiometry (3.7 GHz). The two reasons for using the radiometer at 3.7 GHz are: (i) it works farther away from RFI's due to Wi-Fi and mobile phones, and (ii) it is the protection of the circuit of input radiometer.

The structure of the top view of a dual-mode antenna with inner circular ASA (for radiometry) and outer square ASA (for heating) is shown in Figure 2.31(a). The superstrate is silicone rubber to avoid too much SAR, produced with the contact of the tissue and metallization, and also used for tuning resonance frequency by altering its thickness. Figure 2.31(b) shows the side view of the antenna enclosed within copper housing to decrease RFI. A copper RF choke (quarter-wavelength) is used for providing high impedance to current flow over coaxial feed 2.

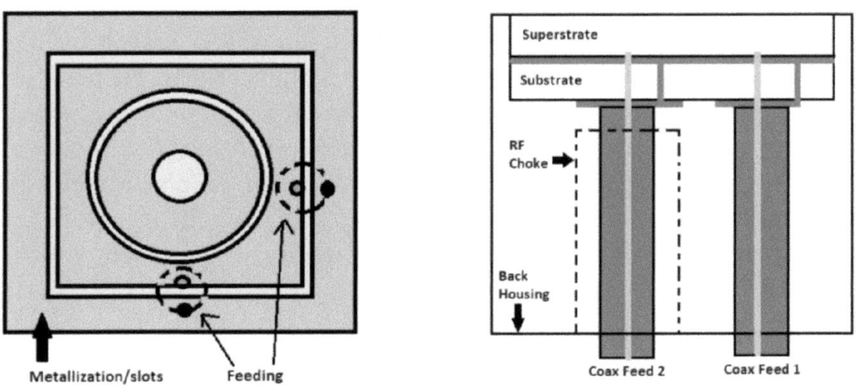

(a) (b)

FIGURE 2.31 (a) Top view of dual mode antenna (b) Side view [19].

For the measurement, a piece of the sponge is positioned inside the beaker filled with saline and allowed the sponge to soak the saline completely. Also, a piece of Teflon sheet or Plexiglas is placed over the sponge as shown in Figure 2.32.

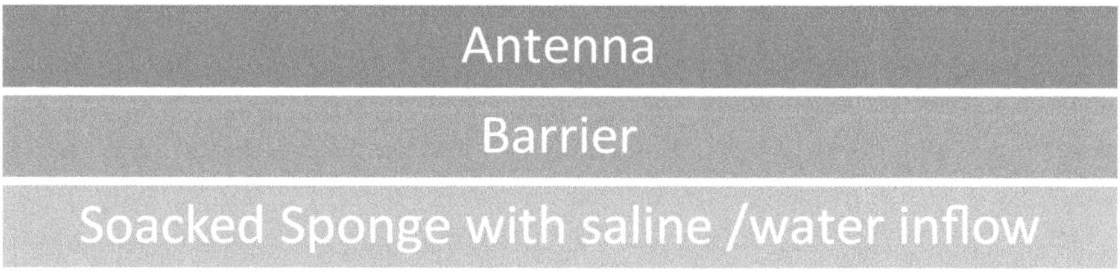

FIGURE 2.32 Soaked sponge in saline [19].

2.7.5 DIFFERENTIALLY FED DUAL-BAND ANTENNA [20]

Early implantable antennas such as microstrip antennas or PIFA were operating at single band frequency. In recent years, dual-band implanted antennas have been introduced to increase the bandwidth. Additionally, triple band and stacked implantable antennas are also introduced. This antenna can be connected to a dual complementary metal oxide semiconductor transmitter for neural signal recording. A superstrate layer is used for protecting antenna from interaction with semiconducting tissue because the superstrate is used as a buffer between tissue and a metal radiator. The antenna has a symmetrical structure and branch having a spiral shape as shown in Figure 2.33, and is connected to the main path to get second resonance. For improved differential circuit connection, the feed is located on the same side of the antenna.

The excitation of the two ports is 180° out of phase and equal in amplitude in the differential feeding. To evaluate the reflection coefficient, the reflection coefficient (odd mode) Γ_{odd} is used, which is given by:

$$\Gamma_{odd} = S_{11} - S_{12} \tag{2.2}$$

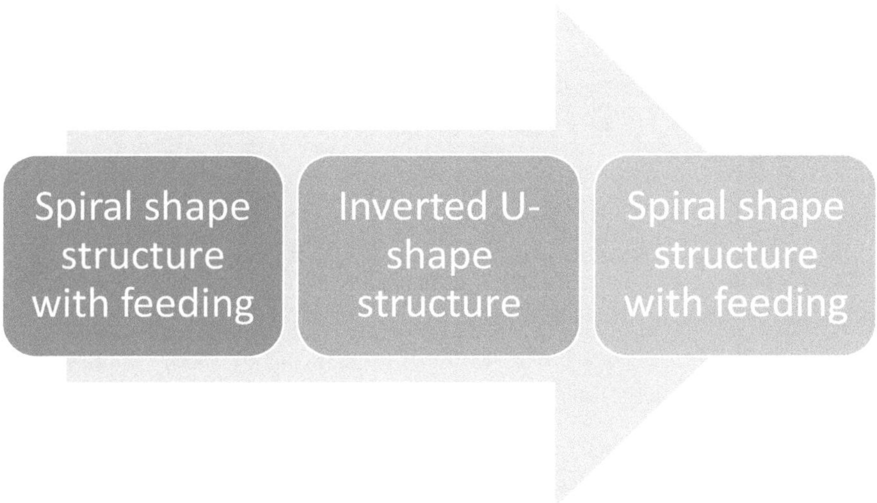

FIGURE 2.33 Structure of differentially fed dual-band antenna [20].

The simulation of this antenna is done with a single-layer and three-layer of tissue. In the single-layer tissue model, the antenna is positioned inside tissue with dimension. The consequence of the position of the antenna in the different layers of tissue is evaluated in the three-layer tissue model. The reflection coefficient (odd mode) does not have variation with the simulation environment. The measurement of this antenna is done using a plastic box filled with tissue-mimicking and skin mimicking gels.

- **Advantages:**
  - It can easily connect to differential circuits.
  - It can eliminate losses produced through the matching circuits and baluns.
- **Application:**
  - Implantable neural recording.

The results of other antennas are presented in Table 2.5.

TABLE 2.5 Other Antennas

Antenna Type	Stacked PIFA [8]	ZOR Antenna [17]	Rectangular Flexible Antenna [18]	Dual-Mode Antenna (Heating) [19]	Differentially Fed Dual Band Antenna [20]	
Year	2012	2011	2017	2016	2012	
Band	MICS	MICS	ISM	nd	MICS	
Volume (mm^3)	nd	328.176	406.78	nd	480.06	
fo (GHz)	0.402	0.402	2.432	0.9	0.4339	0.5424
BW (%/GHz)	0.044	0.009	0.231	nd	7.30%	5.40%
Gain (dBi)	–37.1	–38	4.016	–20.1	nd	nd
SAR 1 g W/Kg	<1.6	1.54/1 g	0.214	nd	0.00244/1 g	0.00266/1 g
PT (mW)	4.927	11.8	2	nd	13.5	
Substrate	Rogers	FR4	Double-sided Rogers	Rogers	Rogers	
Dielectric Constant	10.2	4.4	10.2	3.38	10.2	
Return Loss	>–10	–10	–34	–12.1	>–10	
Simulation Tool	HFSS	nd	CST	HFSS	HFSS	
Model	Anatomical Head Model	Human liquid phantom	Three-layer Skin Model		1 layer and 3 layer tissue model	
In Vitro	Liquid	Liquid	nd	Soaked sponge in saline	Skin Mimicking Gel	
In Vivo	nd	nd	nd	nd	nd	

Note: nd = not defined, BW = bandwidth, PT = input power allowed.

2.8 CONCLUSION

This chapter addresses the overall performance of the different implantable antennas proposed for biomedical applications like pressure monitoring, pacemaker connection, remote health care, real-time measurements, radiometer/heating, checking sugar level, endoscopy, insulin push out, and blood pressure measurement. In accordance with the literature survey, the highest return loss of –45 dB is provided by the textile antenna. The highest impedance bandwidth of 35% is obtained by a dipole antenna with a meander line. The proper value of SAR and maximum input power allowed for patient safety are the main difficult issues, which should be addressed in implantable biomedical antennas.

KEYWORDS

- **annular slot antennas**
- **human tissues phantoms**
- **implantable antenna**
- **in vitro measurement**
- **in vivo measurement**
- **specific absorption rate**

REFERENCES

1. Liu, C., Guo, Y., Liu, X., & Xiao, S., (2016). An integrated on-chip implantable antenna in 0.18 μm CMOS technology for biomedical applications. *IEEE Transactions on Antennas and Propagation, 64*(3), 1167–1172.
2. Lesnik, R., Verhovski, N., Mizrachi, I., Milgrom, B., & Haridim, M., (2018). Gain enhancement of a compact implantable dipole for biomedical applications. *IEEE Antennas and Wireless Propagation Letters, 17*(10), 1778–1782.
3. Adel, D., Hilal, M. E. M., & Soubhi, A. C., (2018). In implantable antennas for biomedical applications: An overview on alternative antenna design methods and challenges. *International Conference on High Performance Computing and Simulation.*
4. Rahaman, M. A., & Delwar, H. Q., (2019). In design and overall performance analysis of an open-end slot feed miniature micro strip antenna for on-body

biomedical applications. *International Conference on Robotics, Electrical, and Signal Processing Techniques (ICREST)* (pp. 200–204). Dhaka, Bangladesh, Dhaka, Bangladesh.
5. Xu, L., Guo, Y., & Wu, W., (2013). Miniaturized slot antenna for biomedical applications. *Electronics Letters, 49*(17), 1060–1061.
6. Scarpello, M. L., et al., (2011). Design of an implantable slot dipole conformal flexible antenna for biomedical applications. *IEEE Transactions on Antennas and Propagation, 59*(10), 3556–3564.
7. Rabbani, M. S., & Ghafouri-Shiraz, H., (2017). Liquid crystalline polymer substrate-based the micro strip antenna arrays for medical applications. *IEEE Antennas and Wireless Propagation Letters, 16*, 1533–1536.
8. Kiourti, A., Costa, J. R., Fernandes, C. A., Santiago, A. G., & Nikita, K. S., (2012). *Miniature Implantable Antennas for Biomedical Telemetry: From Simulation to Realization, 59*(11), 3140–3147.
9. Ashyap, Y. I., et al., (2017). Compact and low-profile textile EBG-based antenna for wearable medical applications. *IEEE Antennas and Wireless Propagation Letters, 16*, 2550–2553.
10. Soh, P. J., et al., (2013). A smart wearable textile array system for biomedical telemetry applications. *IEEE Transactions on Microwave Theory and Techniques, 61*(5), 2253–2261.
11. Liu, C., Guo, Y., & Xiao, S., (2014). Capacitively loaded circularly polarized implantable patch antenna for ISM band biomedical applications. *IEEE Transactions on Antennas and Propagation, 62*(5), 2407–2417.
12. Xu, L., Guo, Y., & Wu, W., (2015). Miniaturized circularly polarized loop antenna for biomedical applications. *IEEE Transactions on Antennas and Propagation, 63*(3), 922–930.
13. Lei, W., Chu, H., & Guo, Y., (2016). Design of a circularly polarized ground radiation antenna for biomedical applications. *IEEE Transactions on Antennas and Propagation, 64*(6), 2535–2540.
14. Li, H., Guo, Y., & Xiao, S., (2016). Broadband circularly polarized implantable antenna for biomedical applications. *Electronics Letters, 52*(7), 504–506.
15. Yang, Z., Xiao, S., Zhu, L., Wang, B., & Tu, H., (2017). A circularly polarized implantable antenna for 2.4-GHz ISM band biomedical applications. *IEEE Antennas and Wireless Propagation Letters, 16*, 2554–2557.
16. Paikhomba, L., & Lakhvinder, S. S., (2017). A brief review on implantable antennas for biomedical applications. *International Journal of Advanced Research in Science and Engineering, 6*(5), 207–222.
17. Ha, J., Kwon, K., & Choi, J., (2011). Compact zeroth-order resonance antenna for implantable biomedical service applications. *Electronics Letter, 47*(23), 1267–1269.
18. Aleef, T. A., Hagos, Y. B., Minh, V. H., Khawaldeh, S., & Pervaiz, U., (2017). Design and simulation-based performance evaluation of a miniaturized implantable antenna for biomedical applications. *Micro and Nano Letters, 12*(10), 821–826.

19. Tofighi, M., & Pardeshi, J. R., (2017). Interference enhanced biomedical antenna for combined heating and radiometry application. *IEEE Antennas and Wireless Propagation Letters, 16*, 1895–1898.
20. Duan, Z., Guo, Y., Xue, R., Je, M., & Kwong, D., (2012). Differentially fed dual-band implantable antenna for biomedical applications. *IEEE Transactions on Antennas and Propagation, 60*(12), 5587–5595.

CHAPTER 3

Biomedical Sensors Using Split Ring Resonators

SUSHMITA BHUSHAN and SANJEEV KUMAR

Department of ECE, Ambedkar Institute of Advanced Communication Technologies and Research, Delhi, India,
E-mails: Sushmita.iert@gmail.com (S. Bhushan), skgaale@gmail.com (S. Kumar)

ABSTRACT

In today's era, sensors are very essential in each and every field like food safety, atmosphere monitoring, disease diagnostics, etc. There are several techniques used for implementing sensors. Few examples of those techniques are surface plasmon resonance, ultrasonic waves, nonmaterial, electrical transducer, etc. But sensors based on these techniques are complex to design, need very sophisticated instruments, and lots of time. In recent years, the metamaterial is widely used in the microwave regime to implement sensors for various applications.

A metamaterial is an artificially designed material that exhibits a negative refractive index (negative permeability and permittivity). Its property depends on its structure and chemical composition. Metamaterials can be designed by making different metallic structures on the substrate like FR4, Roger, etc. These materials are classified into two categories: resonant and non-resonant metamaterial. Split ring resonator (SRR) is a type of resonant metamaterial. In SRR, both permeability and permittivity are negative and have a large varying range. Sensors based on the SRR are very easy to design, cost-effective, very sensitive, and give a quick response. In SRR, the main sensing parameter is its resonant frequency. With the small change in the structure of SRR, a great change in the resonant frequency can occur. In this chapter, we will define the metamaterial, SRR, and defected ground structure (DGS). The theory and structure of SRR will also be discussed in detail with the various application of defected ground SRR as sensors.

3.1 METAMATERIAL

Metamaterials are the artificially constructed materials to obtain the electrical properties which are not available in nature. These materials may consist of periodic or non-periodic structures. The electrical properties of metamaterials depend on their structure and chemical composition. One more important feature of the metamaterial is that the structure size of the material is smaller or equal to the sub-wavelength. Microwave metamaterials are fabricated by designing different metallic structures on a substrate which may be FR4, RT duroid, epoxy, etc. By changing the substrate, we can change the properties of metamaterial. The first experimental left-handed metamaterial represented by Smith et al. [1] is shown in Figure 3.1.

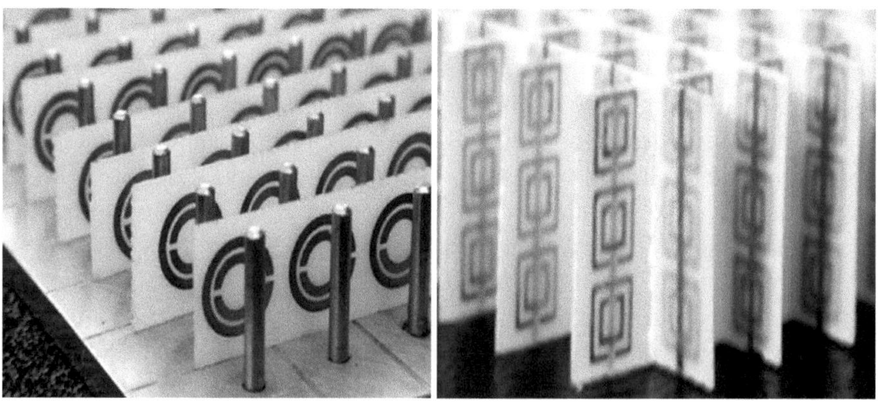

(a) (b)

FIGURE 3.1 The first experimental left-handed metamaterial.

Magnetic permeability and electric permittivity are the characteristics of each material that describes their properties. Metamaterials have negative permittivity and permeability.

3.2 CLASSIFICATION OF METAMATERIALS

According to their properties, metamaterials are classified into two categories:

1. resonant metamaterial; and
2. non-resonant metamaterial.

In the case of resonant metamaterial, a tiny change in resonant frequency can exhibit a huge change in permeability and permittivity. This is the advantage of resonant metamaterials. On the other hand, in the case of non-resonant metamaterials, there is a small change in permittivity and permeability with the small change in frequency. So, the selection of metamaterial design depends on the application of the device.

3.2.1 SPLIT RING RESONATOR

Split ring resonator (SRR) is the type of resonant metamaterial which have negative magnetic permeability. Faraday discovered the diamagnetism theory of closed circuit. When a closed circuit is exposed to an external time-varying magnetic field, the current would be induced in it. Due to this current, secondary magnetic flux is created which is just opposite to the flux and is created by the external magnetic field. This whole process elaborates diamagnetism [2]. However, the negative magnetic permeability cannot be achieved by this effect because the diamagnetic effect of the closed-circuit is not so much strong.

In 1966, a structure is proposed by Schelkunoff, in which a capacitor is loaded on a closed metallic ring to enhance the magnetic permeability [3]. However, this structure is also very difficult to manufacture at the microwave frequencies. To overcome these difficulties at microwave frequencies, Pendry has introduced a structure of SRR in which distributed capacitors are used in place of lumped capacitors [4].

The split ring resonator may have different shapes like circular, square, or triangular. It consists of a ring of metal with a slit or gap on a substrate. A physical model of a split ring resonator is basically consisting of an equivalent LC resonator circuit (Figure 3.2).

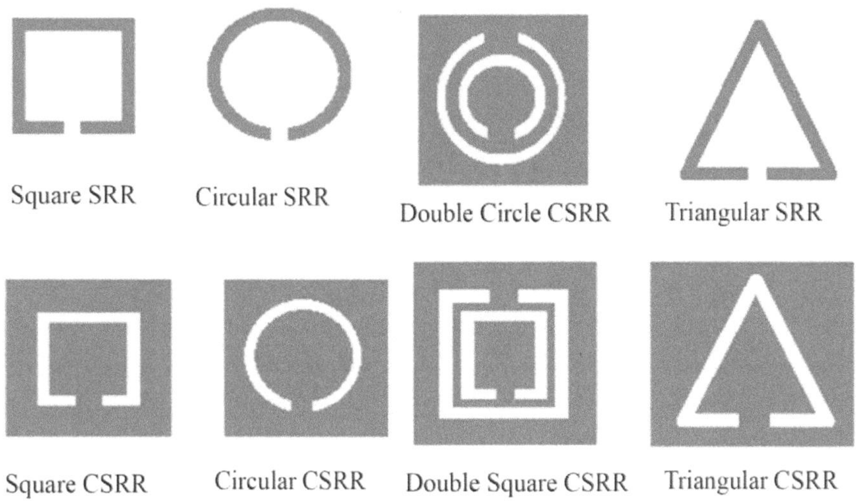

FIGURE 3.2 Types of SRR.

3.2.2 ANALYSIS OF SRR

The SRR consists of a metallic slit ring as shown in Figure 3.3. When a time-varying magnetic field is applied to the SRR, the current starts to flow.

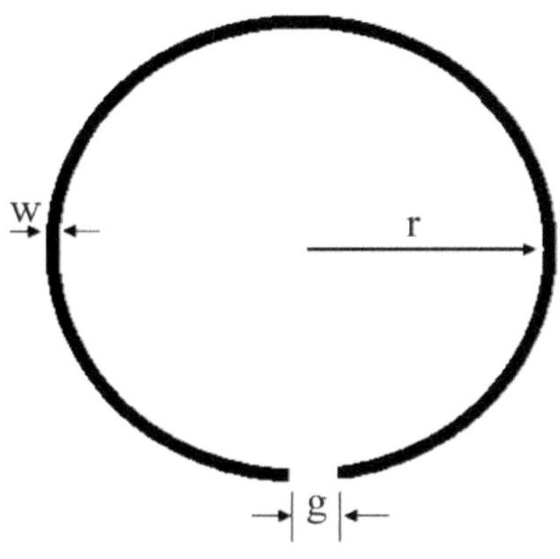

FIGURE 3.3 SRR structure.

An equivalent parallel LC circuit can be used to represent the split ring resonator. Here, the flux associated through the ring is equivalent to inductance L, and the split between the ring is equal to the gap capacitance C. Figure 3.4 explains the equivalent circuit of SRR.

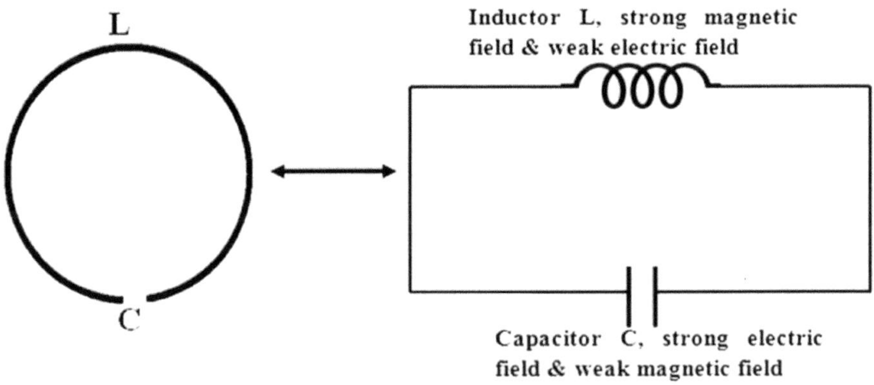

FIGURE 3.4 Equivalent circuit of SRR.

3.3 PARAMETERS OF SRR

Resonant frequency, inductance, and capacitance of a SRR depend on its geometry as shown in Figures 3.5 and 3.6.

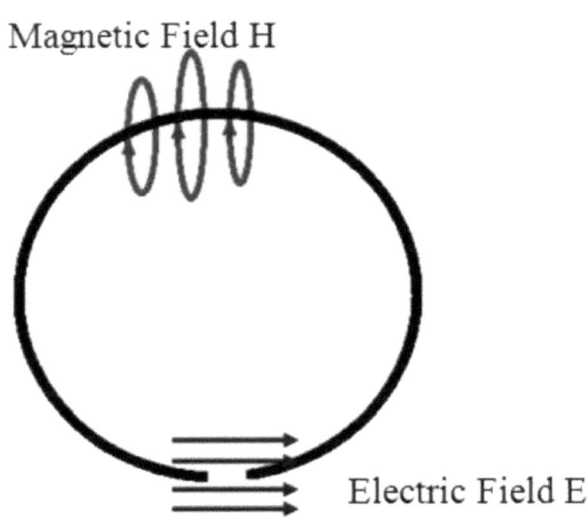

FIGURE 3.5 Schematic of SRR.

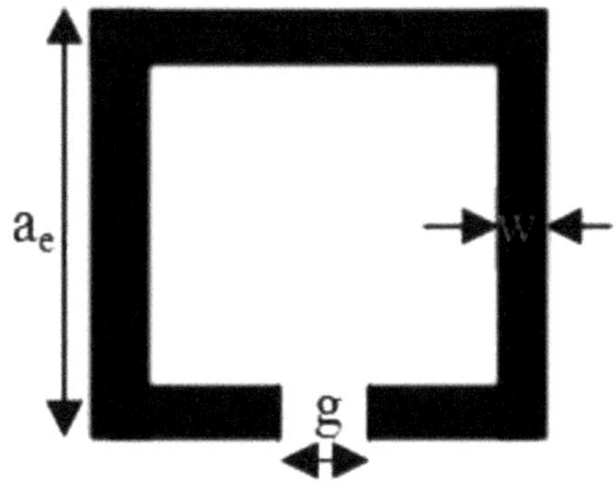

FIGURE 3.6 Geometry of square SRR.

The geometry of the split ring resonator includes the ring's edge dimension (a_e), width of the ring (w), split gap (g), and thickness of metal (h). We can express the resonant frequency of SRR as [5].

$$f_0 = \frac{1}{2\pi\sqrt{L_{net}C_{net}}} \tag{3.1}$$

Here the inductance (L_{net}) and capacitance (C_{net}) depend on the shape of the SRR. The net capacitance of the SRR is the combination of the gap capacitance (C_g) and surface capacitance (C_s). The expression for the gap capacitance and surface capacitance can be stated as follows [6]:

$$C_g = \frac{\varepsilon_0 wt}{g} \tag{3.2}$$

$$C_s = (4a_e - g)C_{pul} \tag{3.3}$$

Here, capacitance per unit length (C_{pul}) can be calculated as:

$$C_{pul} = \frac{\sqrt{\varepsilon_r}}{CZ_0} \tag{3.4}$$

Here, ε_r is the effective permittivity of the medium, C denotes the velocity of light, and Z_0 denotes characteristic impedance of the line. The net inductance can be expressed as [7]:

$$L_{net} \approx \mu_0 l\left[\log\left(\frac{8l}{w+h}\right) - 0.5\right] \tag{3.5}$$

where $L = a_e/2$ and μ_0 is the free space permeability.

3.3.1 SPLIT RING RESONATOR WITH DEFECTED GROUND

In normal SRR design, the SRR is printed on the top side of the substrate and the backside is kept infinite ground. To improve the performance of the SRR sensor, defected ground structure (DGS) is introduced on the bottom side of the substrate. It is observed that by using this structure we can improve the bandwidth and sensitivity of the SRR sensors. SRR size can also be reduced by using the defected ground. To understand the defected ground SRR we have to first understand the theory of DGS.

3.3.2 DEFECTED GROUND STRUCTURE (DGS)

DGS is evolved from the photonic bandgap (PBG) structure. Photonic bandgap structure is also recognized as an electronic band-gap (EBG) structure [8, 9]. DGS works as a low pass filter with a wide band stop. Refs. [10, 11] explain the development of DGS from EBG structure.

As the name suggests, DGS is the periodic or non-periodic structures that are etched from the ground layer of a planer transmission line. Because of these defects, current distribution in the ground plane is disturbed [12–14] and because of this, some transmission line characteristics like capacitance, resistance, and inductance are also changed. With the change in size and shape of the DGS, operating frequency is also changed. In Ref. [15], the first one-dimensional DGS was introduced by Kim et al.

Based on the configuration, DGS can be classified into two categories:

- unit DGS; and
- periodic DGS.

Various shapes of DGS are reported in Refs. [10, 13–21]. These are used in the microwave field to control harmonics, suppress unwanted surface wave, and as a filter. The first dumbbell shape DGS and its response introduced [15] are shown in Figure 3.7.

In periodic DGS, the single DGS unit is repeated at a finite distance. Distance between the DGS unit and their shapes influence the periodic DGS performance. The use of periodic DGS improves the performance and miniaturization can also be achieved. Periodic DGS unit may be arranged in a horizontally and vertically manner as shown in Figure 3.8.

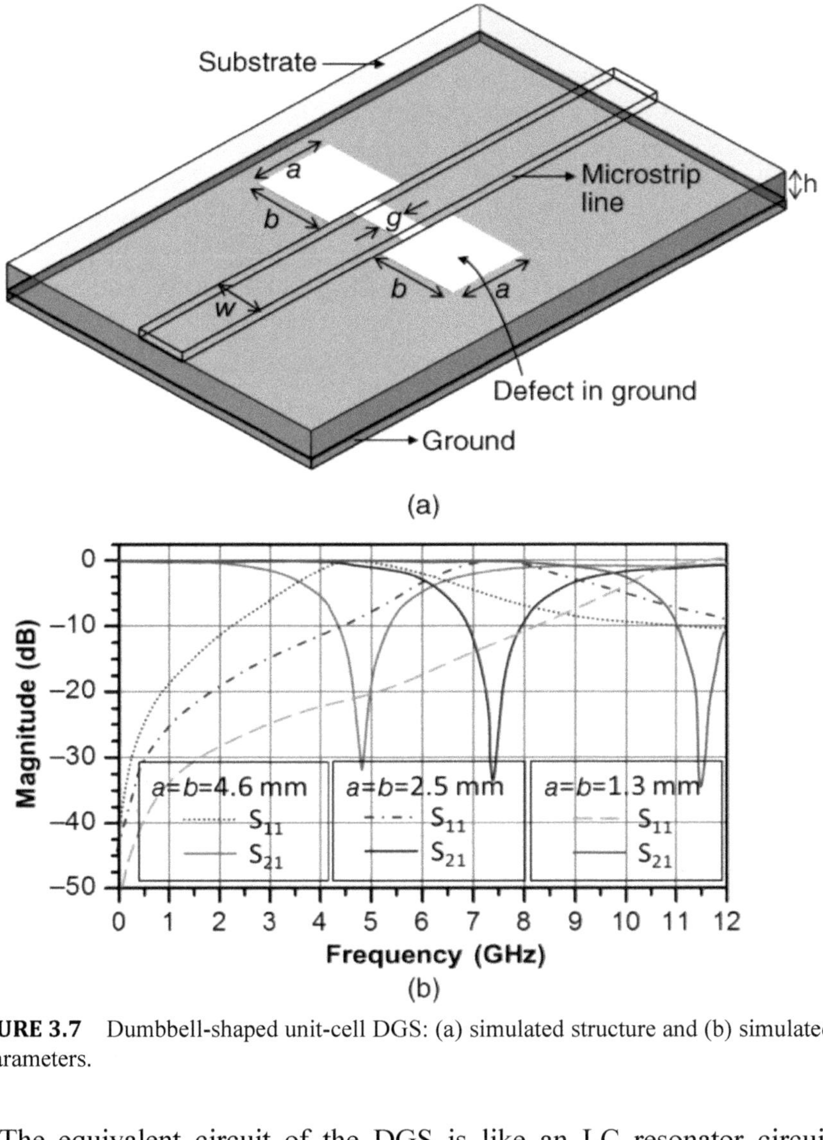

FIGURE 3.7 Dumbbell-shaped unit-cell DGS: (a) simulated structure and (b) simulated S-parameters.

The equivalent circuit of the DGS is like an LC resonator circuit which is coupled to the microstrip line. The shape and size of defects on the ground decide the LC parameter. There are four ways to find out the parameters of the equivalent circuit:

- π shaped equivalent circuit;
- quasi-static equivalent circuit;

- LC and RLC equivalent circuits; and
- using an ideal transformer.

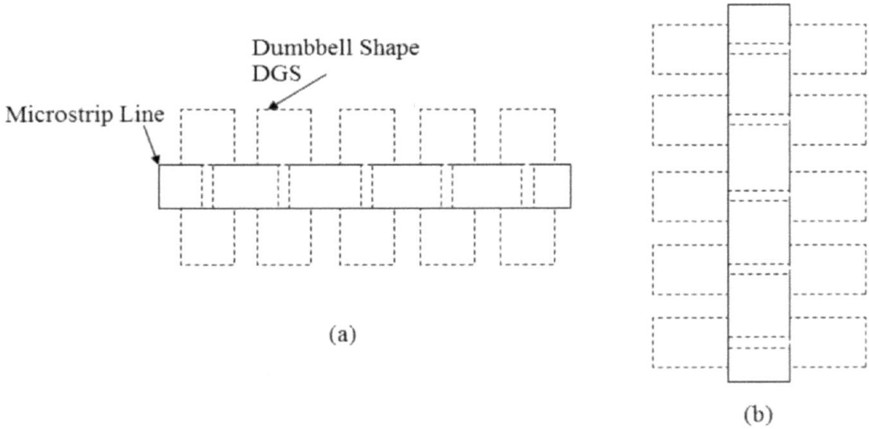

FIGURE 3.8 Periodic DGS: (a) HPDGS; (b) VPDGS.

LC and RLC are the general methods to find out the parameters of DGS. The method for calculating the parameter is given in Ref. [12]. For more accuracy, the RLC model is used which is described in Ref. [22]. The extraction of parameters using quasi-static modeling is described in Ref. [23]. The ideal transformer method for extracting the parameter is given in Ref. [24]. The disadvantage in LC and RLC equivalent circuit is that there is no direct relationship between the L or C and the dimension of defects. This is a time-consuming method and therefore, the quasi-static approach is better than the previous one but this method is complex and the location of the defected structure cannot be obtained. The ideal transformer method is the best one for extracting the parameters and it can determine the location of the defected structure also. DGS has wide applications in microwave circuits and antennas.

3.3.3 APPLICATION OF SRR AS BIOMEDICAL SENSORS

SRR is widely used as a sensor in the biomedical region. The design and fabrication of SRR sensors are very easy. These sensors are very sensitive and give responses very quickly. Some examples of SRR sensors we will discuss here.

3.4 AN ANTENNA COUPLED SPLIT RING RESONATOR FOR BIOSENSING

In this application, an SRR has been used for biosensing applications [5]. Here a metallic ring having a gap is used as an SRR structure on the top layer of the FR4 sheet. The aluminum plate is kept at the bottom to provide grounding. Two microstrip antennas are used to excite the SRR. The SRR resonates at 2.12 GHz frequency. The SRR structure used for this is shown in Figure 3.9.

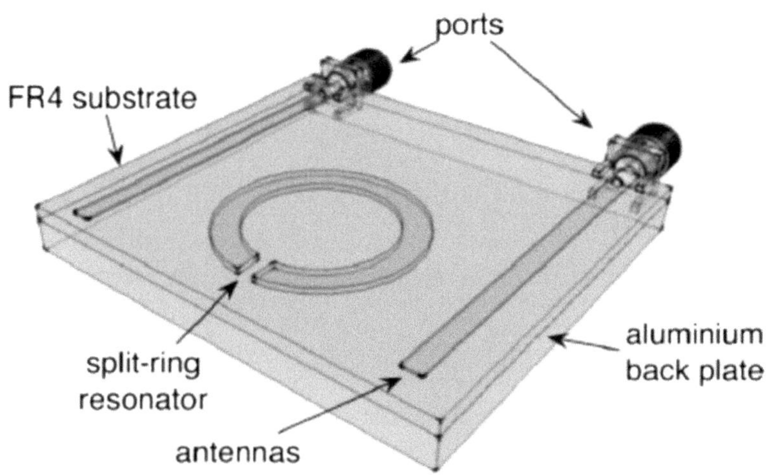

FIGURE 3.9 Antenna coupled SRR for biosensing.

On top of the SRR structure, a layer of parylene is deposited to seal the structure. The characteristic of the SRR is observed by placing different liquid at a different location. Here FGF2 (fibroblast growth factor 2) and heparin are used for biomedical experiments. Shifts in resonant frequency by placing a droplet of the liquids are used for sensing applications. Different location and their responses are shown in Figure 3.10.

3.5 DNA SENSING USING SRR ALONE AT MICROWAVE REGIME

A double split-ring resonator (DSRR) is used for DNA sensing [25]. Sensing of DNA is done by the resonant frequency shifting. The DSRR is excited by the microstrip of 50-ohm characteristic impedance. Figure 3.11 shows the structure of DSRR which is used for DNA sensing.

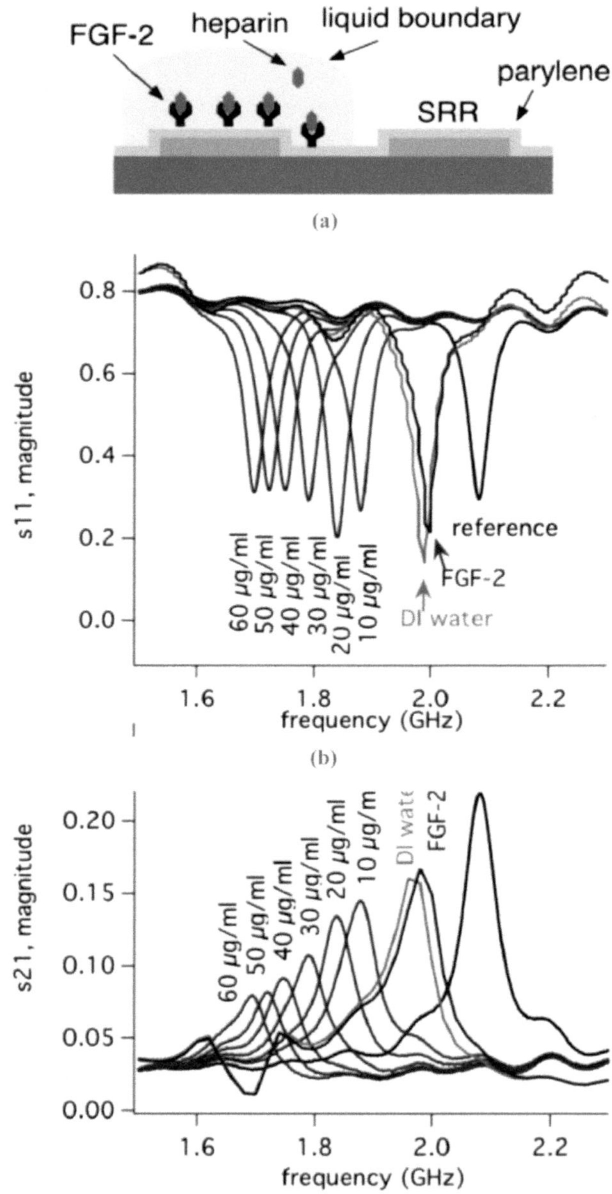

FIGURE 3.10 (a) Schematic of the experimental setup, (b) S11 spectra, and (c) S21 spectra.

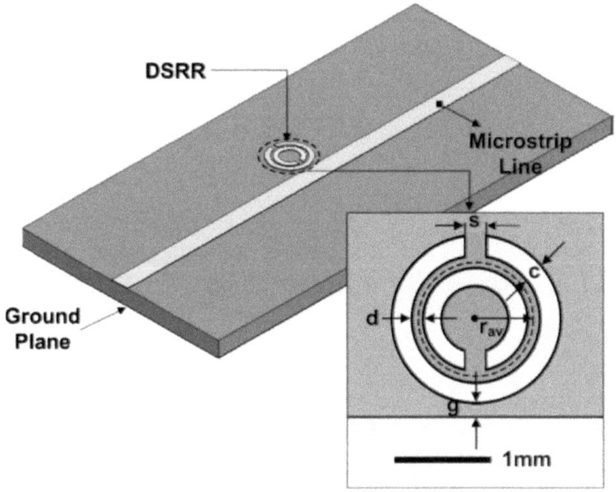

FIGURE 3.11 DSRR sample for DNA sensing (d = 0.1 mm, c = 0.18 mm, s = 0.2 mm, a = 0.68 mm, and g = 0.2 mm).

For the designing of DSRR, a substrate of 0.76 mm thick and having 9.7 dielectric constants is used. To fabricate a biosensing device, a 3 to 5 μm thick layer of Ni and 0.05 μm thick layer of gold are deposited on a copper pattern. The simulated result of DSRR is shown in Figure 3.12. For experimental purposes, single stranded-DNA (ss-DNA), and complementary-DNA (c-DNA) are used as a sensitive element.

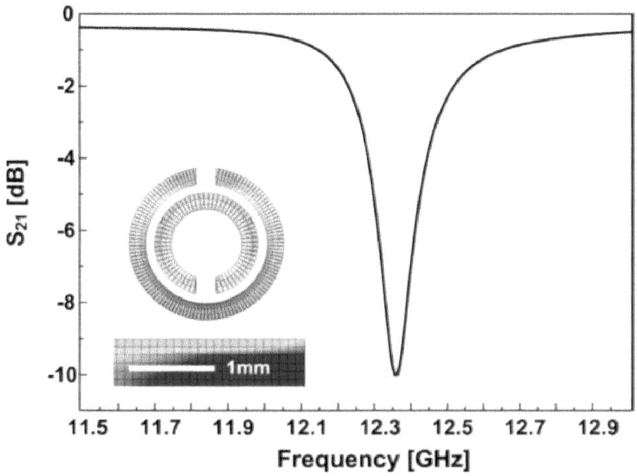

FIGURE 3.12 Simulated result of DSRR.

The measured frequency response of DSRR is shown in Figure 3.13. The resonant frequency of the DSRR is observed 12.35 GHz and is being shifted from 12.35 GHz to 12.33 GHz, when the surface comes into the contact of ss-DNA. After the hybridization of ss-DNA with the c-DNA, frequency has been shifted to 12.27 GHz.

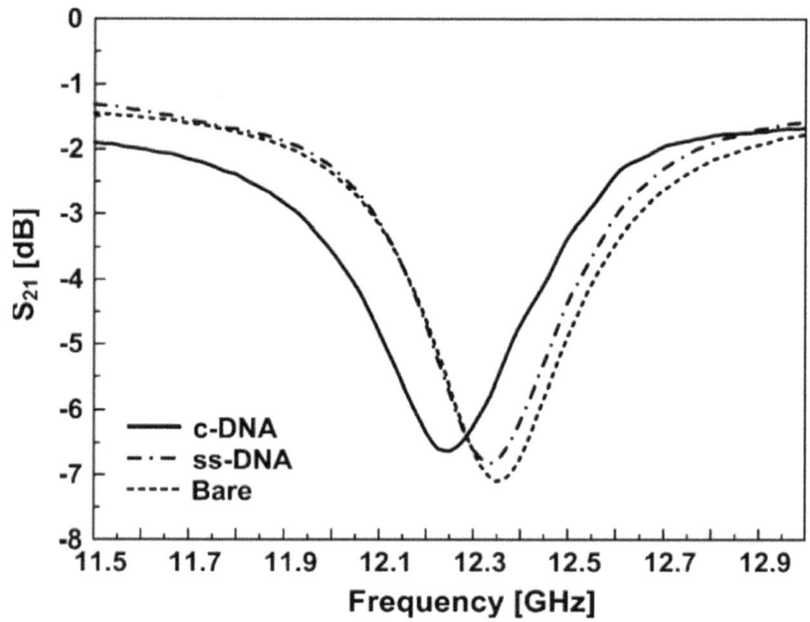

FIGURE 3.13 Measured result of biosensor.

3.6 ASYMMETRIC SRR-BASED BIOSENSOR FOR DETECTION OF LABEL-FREE STRESS BIOMARKERS

In this work, an asymmetric SRR is used as the biosensor for the detection of label-free stress biomarkers [26]. Here, cortisol and alpha(a)-amylase stress biomarkers are used for testing the sensor performance (Figure 3.14).

Here the aSRR is compared with the symmetric SRR (sSRR) and it is observed that the resonance graph of the aSRR is deeper than sSRR. Measured and simulated resonant frequencies of aSRR are 11.25 GHz and 11.27 GHz, respectively. The comparison of aSRR and sSRR is shown in Figure 3.15.

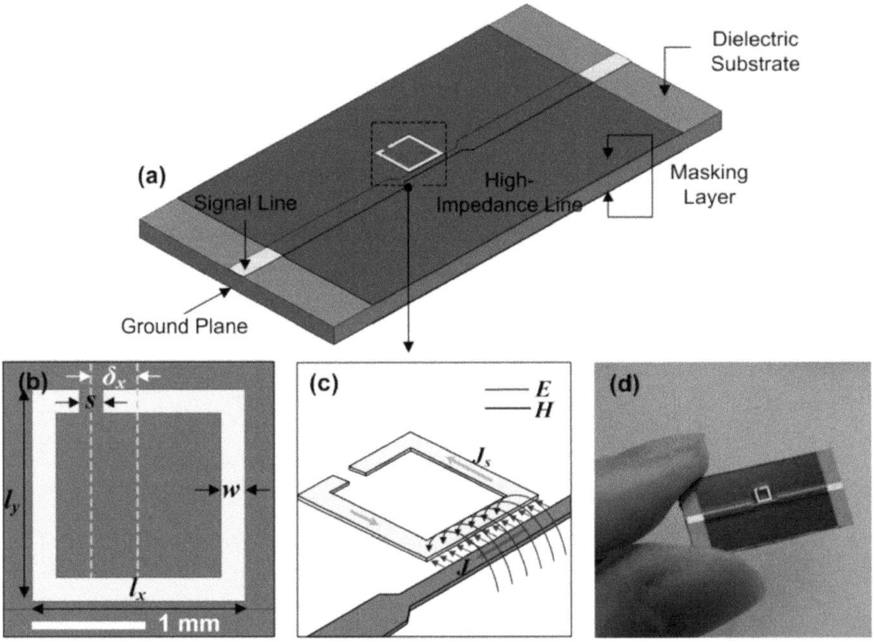

FIGURE 3.14 Schematic and fabricated sample of the sensor.

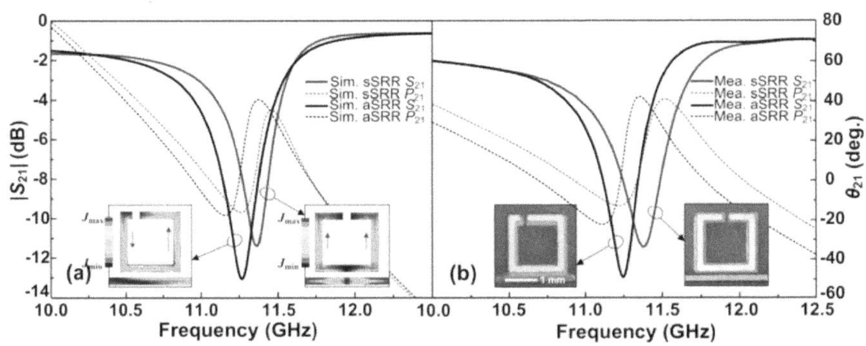

FIGURE 3.15 Comparison between aSRR and sSRR.

3.7 DEFECTED GROUND SRR FOR AN ULTRAFAST SELECTIVE SENSING OF GLUCOSE CONTENT IN BLOOD PLASMA

In this work, an SRR has been designed and fabricated for the testing of glucose content in blood plasma [27]. Here two structures of SRR (i.e., circular and square) are used. The resonant frequency of circular SRR is 1.9 GHz and 8.3 GHz for the square shape SRR.

In this work, DGS is also introduced with the square SRR and it is observed that it provides a sharp cut-off resonant frequency and deep rejection frequency band. The simulated structure of circular SRR and defected ground square SRR are shown in Figure 3.16. Sensing responses of circular SRR and square SRR are shown in Figures 3.17 and 3.18, respectively.

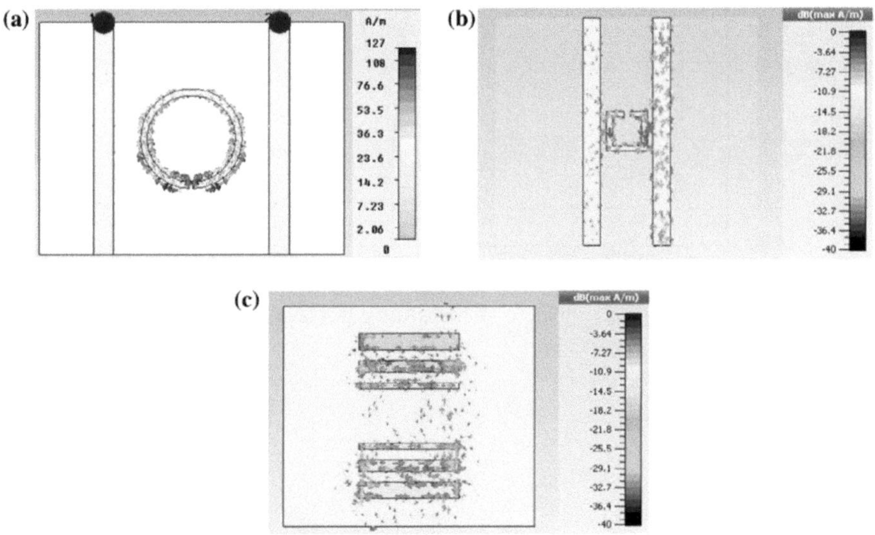

FIGURE 3.16 Simulated structure (a) circular SRR structure (b) square SRR structure.

3.8 SUMMARY

In this chapter, we have introduced the basic concept of metamaterials and split-ring resonators. Designs of sensors based on SRR are also described in this chapter. SRR sensors are very easy to design and use. SRR sensors give a quick and accurate response. It is observed that in the fields of biosensing, SRR sensors are very popular and easy to use. DGS is also introduced with the SRR sensors which enhance the performance of the SRR sensors. Various applications of SRR as biosensors are also discussed in this chapter.

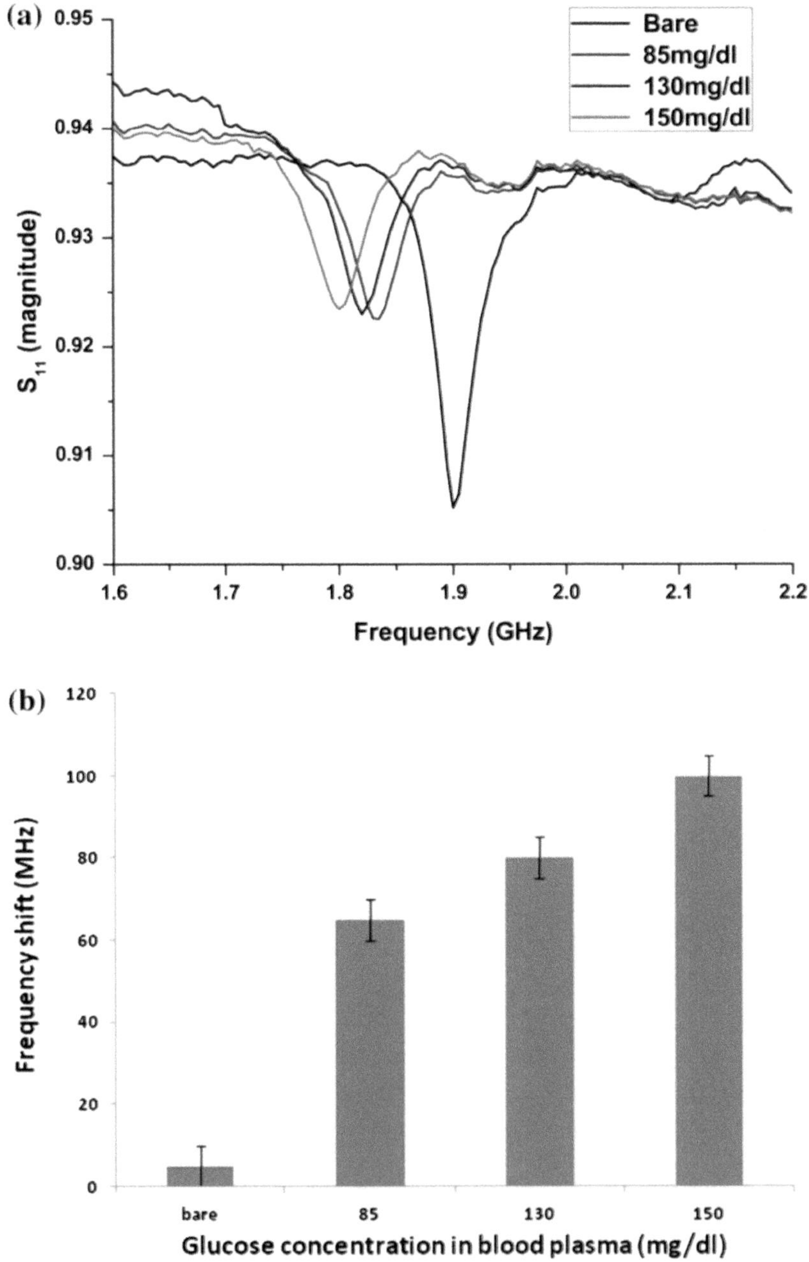

FIGURE 3.17 (a) The frequency response of SRR with different concentrations of glucose in blood plasma, (b) the corresponding frequency shift.

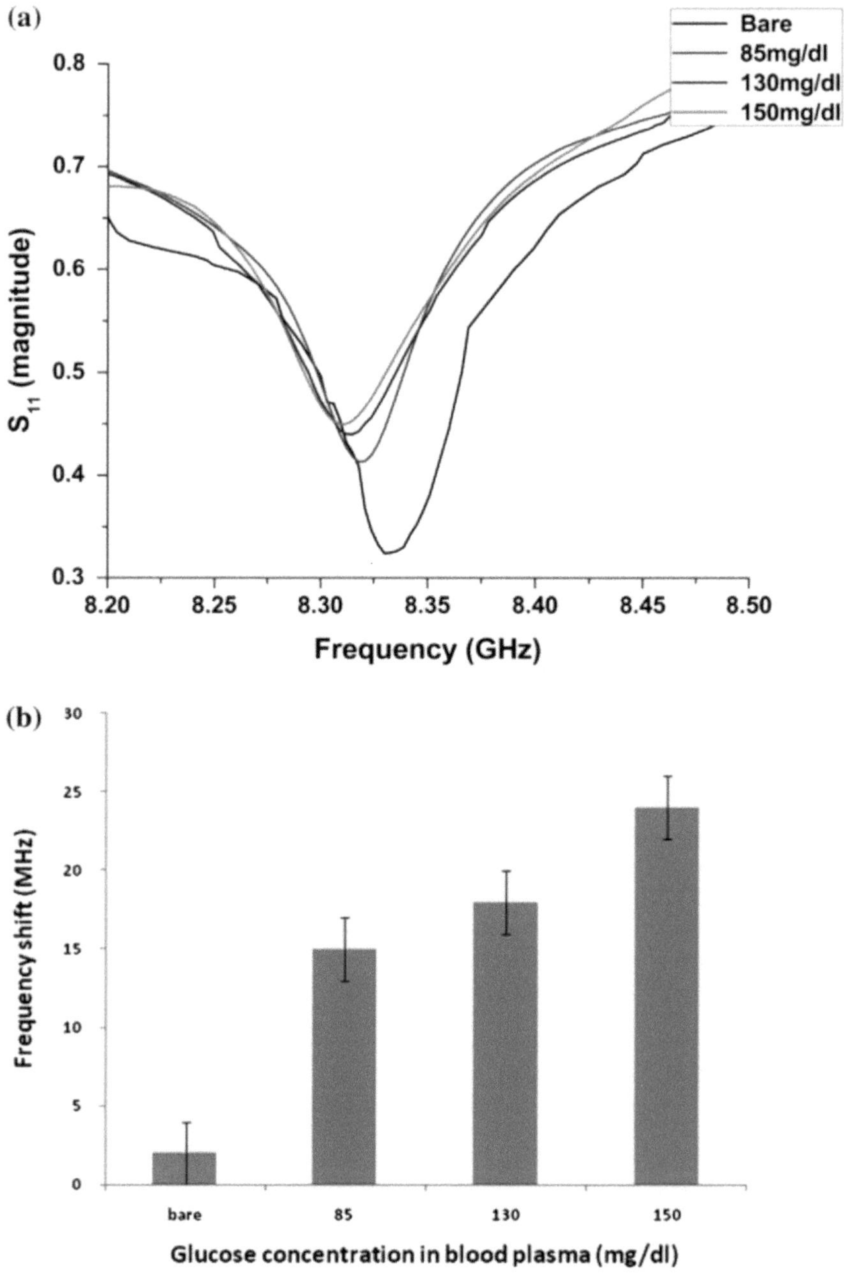

FIGURE 3.18 (a) The frequency response of square SRR with different concentrations of glucose in blood plasma, (b) the corresponding frequency shift.

KEYWORDS

- **defected ground structure**
- **double split-ring resonator**
- **electronic band-gap**
- **photonic band-gap**
- **split ring resonator**
- **symmetric SRR**

REFERENCES

1. Shelby, R. A., Smith, D. R., & Schultz, S., (2001). Experimental verification of a negative index of refraction. *Science, 292*, 77–79.
2. Hayt, W., (1989). *Engineering Electromagnetics* (5th edn.). MC Graw-Hill.
3. Shelkunoff, S. A., & Friis, H. T., (1966). *Antennas Theory and Practice* (3rd edn.). Wiley, New York.
4. Pendry, J. B., Holden, A. J., Robbins, D. J., & Stewart, W. J., (1999). IEEE transactions on microwave theory and techniques. *Magnetism from Conductors and Enhanced Nonlinear Phenomena, 47*(11), 2075–2084.
5. Torun, H., Cagri, T. F., Dundar, G., & Yalcinkaya, A. D., (2014). An antenna-coupled split-ring resonator for bio-sensing. *Journal of Applied Physics*, 116.
6. Selvaraju, R., Jamaluddin, M. H., Kamarudin, M. R., Nasir, J., & Dahri, M. H., (2018). Complementary split ring resonator for isolation enhancement in 5 g communication antenna array. *Progress in Electromagnetics Research C, 83*, 217–228.
7. Sydoruk, O., Tatartschuk, E., Shamonina, E., et al., (2008). Resonant frequency of singly split single ring resonators: An analytical and numerical study. *Presented at Metamaterials' 2008, 2nd International Congress on Advanced Electromagnetic Materials in Microwaves and Optics.* Pamplona, Spain.
8. Dal, A., Jun-Seok, P., Chul-Soo, K., Juno, K., Yongxi, Q., & Itoh, T., (2001). A design of the low-pass filter using the novel micro strip defected ground structure. *IEEE Trans. Microw. Theory Techniq., 49*, 86–93.
9. Yang, F. R., Ma, K. P., Yongxi, Q., & Itoh, T., (1999). A uniplanar compact photonic-band gap (UC-PBG) structure and its applications for microwave circuit. *IEEE Trans. Microw. Theory Techniq., 47*, 1509–1514.
10. Guha, D., Biswas, S., & Antar, Y. M. M., (2010). Defected ground structure for micro strip antennas. In: Guha, D., & Antar, Y. M. M., (eds.), *Micro Strip and Printed Antennas* (pp. 387–343). John Wiley & Sons, Ltd.: New York.
11. Mollah, M. N., Karmakar, N. C., & Fu, J. S., (2005). Investigation of novel tapered hybrid defected ground structure (DGS). *Int. J. RF Microw. Comp. Aided Eng., 15*, 544–550.

12. Ahn, D., Park, J. S., Kim, C. S., Kim, J., Qian, Y., & Itoh, T., (2001). A design of the low-pass filter using the novel micro strip defected ground structure. *IEEE Transactions on Microwave Theory and Techniques, 49*(1), 86–93.
13. Woo, D. J., Lee, T. K., Lee, J. W., Pyo, C. S., & Choi, W. K., (2006). Novel U-slot and V-slot DGSs for band stop filter with improved Q factor. *IEEE Transactions on Microwave Theory and Techniques, 54*(6), 2840–2847.
14. Liu, H. W., Li, Z. F., & Sun, X. W., (2003). A novel fractal defected ground structure and its application to the low-pass filter. *Microwave and Optical Technology Letters, 39*(6), 453–456.
15. Chul-Soo, K., Jun-Seok, P., Dal, A., & Lim, J. B., (2000). A novel 1-D periodic defected ground structure for planar circuits. *IEEE Microw. Guided Wave Lett., 10*, 131–133.
16. Abdel-Rahman, A. B., Verma, A. K., Boutejdar, A., & Omar, A. S., (2004). Control of band stop response of Hi-Lo microstrip low-pass filter using slot in ground plane. *IEEE Trans. Microwave Theory Tech., 52*(3), 1008–1013.
17. Kim, C. S., Lim, J. S., Nam, S., Kang, K. Y., & Ahn, D., (2002). Equivalent circuit modeling of spiral defected ground structure for micro strip line. *Electronic Lett., 38*(19), 1109–1110.
18. Chen, J., Huang, T. H., Chang, C. S., Chen, L. S., Wang, N. F., Wang, Y. H., & Houng, M. P., (2006). A novel cross-shape DGS applied to design ultra-wide stop band low-pass filters. *IEEE Microwave Wireless Components. Lett., 16*(5), 252–254.
19. Mandal, M. K., & Sanyal, S., (2006). A novel defected ground structure for planar circuits. *IEEE Microwave Wireless Components. Lett., 16*(2), 93–95.
20. Burokur, S. N., Latrach, M., & Toutain, S., (2005). A novel type of micro strip coupler utilizing a slot split ring resonators defected ground plane. *Microwave Opt. Technol. Lett., 48*(1), 138–141.
21. Hou, Z. Z., (2008). Novel wideband filter with a transmission zero based on split-ring resonator DGS. *Microwave Opt. Technol. Lett., 50*(6), 1691–1693.
22. Chang, I., & Lee, B., (2002). Design of defected ground structures for harmonic control of active micro strip antenna. *IEEE Antennas and Propagation Society International Symposium, 2*, 852–855.
23. Karmakar, N. C., Roy, S. M., & Balbin, I., (2006). Quasi-static modeling of defected ground structure. *IEEE Trans. Microwave Theory Tech., 54*(5), 2160–2168.
24. Caloz, C., Okabe, H., Iwai, T., & Itoh, T., (2004). A simple and accurate model for micro strip structures with slotted ground plane. *IEEE Microwave Wireless Components. Lett., 14*(4), 133–135.
25. Hee-Jo, L., & Hyun-Seok, L., & Kyung-Hwa, Y., & Jong-Gwan, Y., (2010). DNA sensing using split-ring resonator alone at microwave regime. *Journal of Applied Physics, 108*, 014908–014908. doi: 10.1063/1.3459877.
26. Hee-Jo, L., Jung-Hyun, L., Suji, C., Ik-Soon, J., & Jong-Soon, C., (2013). Asymmetric split-ring resonator-based biosensor for detection of label-free stress biomarkers. *Applied Physics Letters,* 103.
27. Ankita, V., Sushmita, B., Pramod, N. T., Manish, G., & Singh, B. R., (2017). A defected ground split ring resonator for an ultra-fast, selective sensing of glucose content in blood plasma. *Journal of Electromagnetic Waves and Applications, 31*(10), 1049–1061.

CHAPTER 4

Evaluation of Software Fault Proneness with a Support Vector Machine and Biomedical Applications

RENU DALAL,[1] MANJU KHARI,[1] and DIMPLE CHANDRA[2]

[1]*Assistant Professor, Computer Science and Engineering Department, AIACT&R, GGSIPU, Delhi, India, E-mails: dalalrenu1987@gmail.com (R. Dalal), manjukhari@yahoo.co.in (M. Khari)*

[2]*Assistant Professor, Computer Science and Engineering Department, NIET, Greater Noida, Uttar Pradesh, India, E-mail: dimplechandra1988@gmail.com*

ABSTRACT

The high throughput and good quality software are developed if effective defect prone modules can be predicted by testers at early stages. This enables the testers to focus on the activities, allocation of effort, and efficient resource management. Accurate prediction of fault inclined modules in software development manner allows effective detection and identity of defects. The existing researches used support vector machine (SVM) in standalone mode in the sense that no pre-processing is performed before invoking classification; thus degrading the accuracy of prediction. This chapter delivered a singular approach combining SVM and feature choice for software fault proneness prediction (SFPP). Experiments suggest that the accuracy of the proposed method using five object-oriented (OO) metrics, that is, line of code (LOC), program level (L), branch count (BR), and unique operands. Hence, the OO metrics have a large prone in defect prone modules.

4.1 SOFTWARE FAULT PRONENESS WITH SVM

SFPP is a critical undertaking for minimizing cost and improving the general effectiveness of the checking out method [14]. It is widely diagnosed that figuring out and doing away with high-danger problems in software projects have to be performed in software verification and validation [7]. Even though trying out can be targeted on a subset of software program components, it is regularly accomplished primarily based on software metrics, which provide quantitative descriptions of application attributes to degree software fault proneness [47]. Various existing works were proposed to pick out the software program metrics based totally on device gaining knowledge of strategies along with statistical algorithms, choice trees, neural networks, and many others (see Section 4.2 for detail) [15]. However, for the reason that courting among software metrics and fault proneness is often complex, one's metrics cannot be interpreted in phrases of software traits [29]. Thus, a non-linear model inclusive of the support vector machine (SVM) should be used to address the drawback [1].

SVM is a useful method for facts type [6]. It makes use of primary danger minimization criteria for preparing to get to know gadgets and has a decent potential to study and sum up especially [22]. It has been validated that SVM has many unique advantages in fixing small samples, nonlinear, and high-dimensional sample recognition problems [31]. In SVM, kernel functions are used to convert linear fashions to non-linear ones through dot merchandise. The nonlinear SVM maps the education samples from the input area into a better-dimensional function area via a mapping function [25]. SVM then finds a linear setting apart hyperplane with the maximal margin on this dimensional area. Using a radial basis function (RBF) as a kernel, smoother decision surface, and extra normal decision boundary may be decided [24].

In machine learning (ML), guide-vector machines (SVMs) are supervised gaining knowledge of models with related learning algorithms that examine statistics used for classification and regression analysis. SVM attempts to categorize instances by finding a separating boundary known as hyper-aircraft. The main gain of the SVM is that it is able to (with relative ease) conquer 'the high dimensionality hassle;' that is, the trouble that arises while there may be a big wide variety of enter variables relative to the quantity observations. Due to SVM, the technique is statistics-pushed and feasible without a theoretical framework; it may have critical discriminative strength for class, particularly in cases where sample sizes are small. This method is used to enhance techniques for detecting sicknesses in clinical settings. Moreover, SVM has established high overall performance in solving type problems in bioinformatics.

4.1.1 BIOMEDICAL APPLICATIONS OF SVM

- **Recognizing Diseases and Diagnosis:** One of the central ML applications in social insurance is the ID and analysis of illnesses and infirmities, which are generally viewed as difficult to-analyze. This can incorporate anything from tumors, which are hard to find during the underlying stages, to other hereditary illnesses.
- **Medication Discovery and Medicine:** One of the essential clinical uses of SVM lies in the beginning period sedate revelation process. This likewise incorporates R&D innovations, for example, cutting edge sequencing, and accuracy prescription which can help in discovering elective ways for the treatment of multi-factorial sicknesses.
- **Customized Medicine:** Personalized medications matching individual wellbeing with the prescient examination is additionally ready are for further research and better infection appraisal. As of now, doctors are restricted to browsing a particular arrangement of conclusions or gauge the hazard to the patient dependent on his symptomatic history and accessible hereditary data. Nevertheless, AI in the drug is making incredible steps. The results acquired from best in class calculations as if SVM has demonstrated incredible guarantee in customized medication.
- **Clinical Trial and Research:** SVM has a few potential applications in the field of clinical preliminaries and research. Clinical preliminaries cost a great deal of time and cash and can take a very long time to finish as a rule. Applying ML-based prescient examination to recognize potential clinical preliminary, competitors can enable specialists to draw a pool from a wide assortment of information; for example, past specialist visits, online life, and so on.
- **Outbreak Prediction:** Today, researchers approach a lot of information gathered from satellites, continuous web-based social

networking refreshes, site data, and so forth. Calculations like SVM help to order this data and foresee everything from malarial outbreaks to extreme incessant irresistible infections. Anticipating these outbreaks is particularly useful in underdeveloped nations, as they need a critical restorative foundation and instructive frameworks. An essential case of this is the ProMED-mail, an Internet-based detailing stage that screens developing sicknesses and rising ones and gives outbreak reports progressively [24].

It is really worth noting from the present studies that SVM was used in the standalone mode this means that no pre-processing has been achieved with the dataset before invoking category; as a consequence degrading the accuracy of prediction [15]. In this bankruptcy, we propose a new method combining SVM and feature choice for this mission. The SVM is better the usage of information normalization and a characteristic subset choice method like F-score. By doing so, we can specify the maximum crucial functions for a class of illness susceptible modules in SFPP. The kernel choice makes use of the RBF kernel because (i) kernels non-linearly map samples into a higher dimensional space so that RBF, in contrast to the linear kernel, can take care of the case while the relation among elegance labels and attributes is nonlinear; (ii) The variety of hyper aircraft parameters, which influences the complexity of model selection, is various. The polynomial kernel has extra hyper-aircraft parameters than the RBF kernel [2].

The rest of the chapter is organized as follows. Section 4.3 introduces the associated study on SFPP. Section 4.4 confirms the proposed work, facts descriptions; all object-oriented metrics, and four distinct procedures of SVM with distinctive flowcharts. Experimental effects are given in Section 4.4 including graphical representations of character techniques. Finally, end with a precise of the general paintings, and the troubles discovered inside the implementation of the investigated work is highlighted in Section 4.5.

4.2 STUDY ON SOFTWARE FAULT PRONENESS PREDICTION

Applying gadget gaining knowledge of software program fault proneness prediction determined the correlation between some software program metrics and fault proneness has ended in a variety of predictive fashions based totally on a couple of metrics [6]. Guo, Ma, Cukic, and Singh [18] supplied a way for predicting fault-prone modules based totally on random forests (RF) and carried out it in five case researches on NASA datasets. The prediction accuracy of the proposed methodology is normally higher than those completed via logistic regression and discriminant analysis. The universal accuracy is between 75% to 94%, and the disorder detection price is up to 87%. Exhaustive and heuristic search tactics had been carried out for studying a software program defect prediction model. Chen and Cheng [8] defected software program modules cause software program screw-ups, growth improvement, and protection costs, and decrease patron pleasure. The authors proposed a modified minimize entropy principle approach and expand a changed system to partition the data, and then construct the category tree version. Pendharkar [36] proposed a software defect prediction version which is combinatorial optimization trouble with factorial complexity, and hybrid exhaustive searches and probabilistic neural network and simulated annealing tactics to remedy it. The authors in comparison their performance with the conventional class algorithms.

Kumar and Duraisamy [27] evaluated three symmetric ensemble strategies: bagging, boosting, and stacking to predict faulty modules based on evaluating the performance of 11 base beginners. Ma et al. [33] constructed multivariate prediction models to look at the usefulness of network measures underneath three prediction settings: pass-validation, throughout-launch, and inter-undertaking predictions. Singh, Pal, Verma, and Vyas [39] developed a framework for automated extraction of human-comprehensible fuzzy rules for software fault detection/classification. This is an incorporated framework to simultaneously discover beneficial determinants (attributes) of faults and fuzzy guidelines the usage of those attributes. Xiao proposed [44] a recurrent neural community model based totally on a mixture of the echo country network and the dynamic Bayesian network together with a graph-based echo kingdom community and an inference algorithm according to Bayesian policies and probability graph principle. Xu, Gondra, and Chiu [45] aimed toward identifying the underlying concept from collectively categorized facts. Lahsasna and Seng [28] proposed editions of the fuzzy classifier, which are capable of finding more non-dominated fuzzy rule-based structures with better generalization potential than the unique method. Wulf and Bertschn [43] proposed an idea for the era of textual causes for a multi-dimensional preferential sensitivity evaluation, which is particularly beneficial for tough interpretational responsibilities.

Regarding the works using the SVM method, Elish and Elish [12] used this set of rules for predicting illness-inclined software modules towards eight compared models in the context of four NASA datasets. Gondra [14] focused on the way to pick out the software program metrics which can be maximum likely to signify fault proneness. Specifically, given NASA statistics on software program metric values and a variety of suggested mistakes, the authors carried out a comparative experimental examination of neural networks and SVM on a dataset obtained from NASA's metrics data program (MDP) data repository. Arisholm, Briand, and Fuglerud [5] performed an industrial setting that attempts to build predictive fashions to perceive elements of a Java device with a high fault probability. Data mining strategies had been used to evaluate illness proneness modules inclusive of logistic regression, neural community, SVM, boosting, etc. Other works on software program fault proneness prediction may be visible in Refs. [3, 4, 10, 11, 13, 16, 19–21, 23, 24, 30, 32, 35, 37, 38, 40, 46, 48, 49].

4.3 THE PROPOSED METHOD

We realized that the existing methods used SVM in standalone mode that means no pre-processing is done with the dataset before invoking classification; thus degrading the accuracy of prediction [15]. In this section, a novel method combining SVM and feature selection is introduced.

A vital hassle regarding software metrics (e.g., line of code: LOC) is that the top bound of cost range is commonly limitless [37]. It is a common place to estimate the ones bounds from the variety of values determined within the dataset. Hence, our idea of normalizing the facts is accomplished. Because of these normalized values, the computation of similar steps is minimized.

Feature choice (additionally referred to as subset selection) is a technique commonly used in machine mastering, in which subsets of the capabilities available from the data are selected for software of gaining knowledge of the algorithm [34]. The best subset incorporates the least quantity of dimensions that generally contribute to accuracy; we discard the final and unimportant dimensions. This is an important degree of preprocessing and is one among two methods of averting the curse of dimensionality (the other is characteristic extraction) [17]. By disposing of the maximum irrelevant and redundant functions from the statistics, characteristic choice facilitates improving the overall performance of gaining knowledge of models. It additionally helps to obtain higher knowledge of information by using figuring out the maximum important functions and how they may be related to every other. The quality feature choice is the F-score method [41]. Before making use of any fault-proneness method, we observe the F-score characteristic subset selection approach to the input dataset to cast off redundant capabilities. In addition to the proper parameters placing, feature subset choice can improve classification accuracy. If the F-rating value of any feature in the dataset is larger than the imply fee, that feature will be selected. Otherwise, it's far eliminated from the characteristic space. The inappropriate or redundant features are then removed from the enter function area [8].

Eventually, SVM is stronger in the usage of data normalization and in a function choice method (i.e., F-score). By doing so, we can specify the maximum vital functions for a class of disorder prone modules. The hybrid SVM process is given in next Section 4.4.1, and Section 4.3 presents four new techniques of facts normalization and F-rating implemented to the hybrid SVM. In order to recognize the technique, a numerical instance from the NASA records [8] is hooked up to the set of rules.

4.3.1 THE HYBRID SVM METHOD

- **Step 1:** Select the JM1 dataset from the NASA IV & V facility MDP facts repository. The primary goal of the MDP is to acquire, validate, organize, shop, and deliver software program metrics facts.
- **Step 2:** Retrieve and modules which clearly contain complex choice structures. N is the Halstead application duration (N = N1 + N2), V is the Halstead software extent (V = N*log2(n1 + n2)), and L is the Halstead program stage.
- **Step 3:** Normalized the dataset:

$$z_i' = \frac{z_i - \min(z_i)}{\max(z_i) - \min(z_i)} \tag{4.1}$$

In which min (z_i) and max (z_i) are the minimum and most values, respectively, of the ith issue (i.e., software program metric) over the *n* observations within a small subset of the unique dataset (Table 4.1) in which LOC represents for the whole number of strains; V(G) is the quantity of linearly independent paths that measures the complexity of modules choice structure; EV(G) measures how lots unstructured common sense exists in a module; IV(G)-derived from V(G) measures the complexity of a module calling styles as compared to other modules. It differentiates between modules that increase an application design complexity in the dataset. Thus, each recorded fee is mapped to the closed interval [0, 1] as proven in Table 4.2.

TABLE 4.1 Small Subset of JM1 Dataset

LOC	V(G)	EV(G)	IV(G)	N	V	L
1.1	1.4	1.4	1.4	1.3	1.3	1.3
1	1	1	1	1	1	1
72	7	1	6	198	1134.13	0.05
190	3	1	3	600	4348.76	0.06
37	4	1	4	126	599.12	0.06
31	2	1	2	111	582.52	0.08
78	9	5	4	0	0	0
8	1	1	1	16	50.72	0.36
24	2	1	2	0	0	0
143	22	20	10	0	0	0
73	10	4	6	0	0	0
83	11	10	7	0	0	0
12	3	1	1	37	167.37	0.15
48	4	1	4	129	695.61	0.06
68	8	1	5	0	0	0
138	22	10	8	0	0	0
10	1	1	1	9	27	0.5
250	49	34	16	1469	9673.31	0.01
77	8	1	1	284	1160.84	0.02
85	9	1	7	277	1714.58	0.03
110	17	13	8	322	2069.26	0.03
49	6	6	3	171	927.89	0.04
187	35	26	16	526	3296.33	0.02
27	6	6	3	0	0	0
38	8	1	3	145	673.36	0.05
294	43	33	24	814	5811.59	0.02
29	3	1	3	88	465.12	0.08
160	5	4	3	698	4862.12	0.03
94	16	9	5	218	1236.59	0.03

- **Step 4:** (F-score feature subset choice). F-score measures the distinction between two lessons with real values. F-rating values of each function are computed, and then as a way to pick out features from the whole dataset, a threshold price is obtained by using calculating the common cost of F-ratings of all functions as follows.

$$F(i) = \frac{(\bar{z}_i^{(+)} - \bar{z}_i)^2 + (\bar{z}_i^{(-)} - \bar{z}_i)^2}{\frac{1}{n_+ - 1}\sum_{k=1}^{n_+}(\bar{z}_{k,i}^{(+)} - \bar{z}_i^{(+)})^2 + \frac{1}{n_- - 1}\sum_{k=1}^{n_-}(\bar{z}_{k,i}^{(-)} - \bar{z}_i^{(-)})^2} \tag{4.2}$$

TABLE 4.2 Normalized Dataset

LOC	V(G)	EV(G)	IV(G)	N	V	L
2.90613E-05	0	0.002	0.0009975	0	1.6081E-05	1
0	0	0	0	0	1.237E-05	0.769
0.020633537	0	0	0.0124688	0.02	0.01402878	0.038
0.054925894	0	0	0.0049875	0.07	0.05379361	0.046
0.010462075	0	0	0.0074813	0.01	0.0074109	0.046
0.008718396	0	0	0.0024938	0.01	0.00720556	0.062
0.022377216	0	0.024	0.0074813	0	0	0
0.002034292	0	0	0	0	0.00062739	0.277
0.006684103	0	0	0.0024938	0	0	0
0.041267074	0	0.116	0.0224439	0	0	0
0.02092415	0	0.018	0.0124688	0	0	0
0.023830282	0	0.055	0.0149626	0	0	0
0.003196745	0	0	0	0	0.00207031	0.115
0.01365882	0	0	0.0074813	0.02	0.00860445	0.046
0.019471084	0	0	0.0099751	0	0	0
0.039814008	0	0.05	0.0174564	0	0	0
0.002615519	0	0	0	0	0.00033398	0.385
0.072362685	0.1	0.201	0.0374065	0.17	0.11965539	0.88
0.022086603	0	0	0	0.03	0.01435918	0.015
0.024411508	0	0	0.0149626	0.03	0.02120874	0.023
0.0317676838	0	0.073	0.0174564	0.04	0.02559601	0.023
0.013949433	0	0.03	0.0049875	0.02	0.01147767	0.031
0.054054054	0.1	0.152	0.0374065	0.06	0.0407744	0.015
0.007555943	0	0.03	0.0049875	0	0	0
0.010752688	0	0	0.0573566	0.02	0.00832922	0.038
0.085149666	1	0.195	0.0049875	0.1	0.07188729	0.015
0.008137169	0	0	0.0049875	0.01	0.00575337	0.062
0.046207498	0	0.018	0.0049875	0.08	0.06014269	0.023
0.027027027	0	0.049	0.0099751	0.03	0.01529618	0.023

- **Step 5:** Applying the F-score to the original dataset in Table 4.1. Follow Step 7 to find the F-score which is sorted in the ascending order as shown in Table 4.3.

TABLE 4.3 F-Score in Ascending Order of the Original JM1 Dataset

Metric	F-Score
L	0.076905
LOC	0.070321
Branch count	0.05806
I	0.056802
Unique operand	0.052476
IO blank	0.051439
Total operand	0.05112
N	0.05039
Total operator	0.048428
V(G)	0.047723
D	0.44251
IO code	0.42309
EV(G)	0.04179
B	0.039343
V	0.039246
IV(G)	0.034936
IO comment	0.033997
Unique operator	0.031786
IO code & comment	0.016886
T	0.006686
E	0.006686

- **Step 6:** Applying the F-score to the normalized dataset in Table 4.1. Follow Step 7 to find the F-score which is sorted in the ascending order shown in Table 4.4.
- **Step 7:** The procedure is as follows:
  i. Calculate F-score for each function.
  ii. Sort F-score, and set a viable quantity of functions through $f = \left[n/_{2^i} \right], i \in \{0,1,2,\ldots\ldots,m\}$, in which m is an integer with $n/_{2^m} \geq 1$.

iii. For each *f* (threshold), do the subsequent:
   a. Keep the first *f* feature in step with the F-rating.
   b. Randomly cut up the education records into $D_{training}$ and $D_{validation}$ using five-fold cross-validation.
   c. Do the subsequent step for every fold: Let $D_{training}$ is the new training information. Use the SVM system as a predictor; use the predictor to predict $D_{validation}$. Calculate the common validation errors of the five-fold cross-validation.

iv. Choose the *f* (threshold) with the lowest average validation mistakes.

v. Drop features with F-rating beneath the chosen threshold.

- **Step 8:** Apply SVM with "Radial Kernel" on $n/2^m \geq 1$

TABLE 4.4 F-Score in Ascending Order of Normalized JM1 Dataset

F-Score	Metric
0.052864	LOC
0.052465	I
0.046381	Branch count
0.044847	L
0.040764	IO blank
0.040459	N
0.039844	V(G)
0.039224	Total operator
0.038273	Unique operand
0.037252	Total operand
0.035364	EV(G)
0.035072	IO code
0.034207	B
0.034123	V
0.030881	IV(G)
0.029979	IO comment
0.02792	D
0.016763	Unique operator
0.015975	IO code and comment
0.006592	T
0.006592	E

4.3.2 PROPOSED STRATEGIES

The hybrid SVM implementation is greater the use of four distinct strategies as in Figure 4.1. The JM1 dataset is randomized 20 instances, and the SVM prediction is carried out to all 20 particular units that are further divided into the schooling and testing units. True negative (TN), false negative (FN), false positive (FP), and true positive (TP) are taken from the confusion matrix. In 20 distinct JM1 datasets, the kernel parameters and quantity of metrics are constant. Indeed, now examine the effects and take average accuracy and precision.

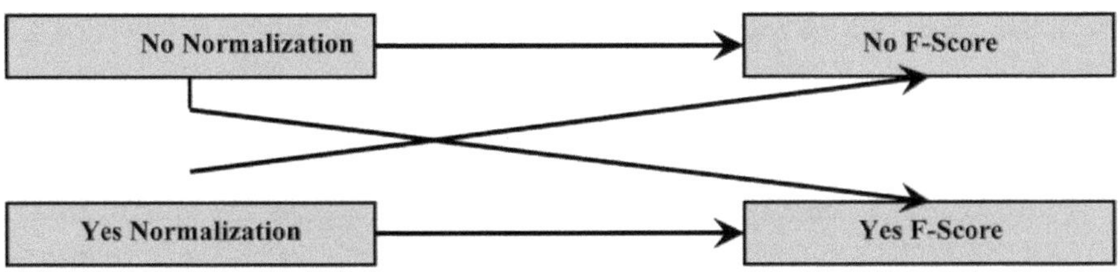

FIGURE 4.1 Pre-processing strategies for SVM prediction.

- **Case 1: No Normalization-No F-Score:** Here the SVM is applied to the original JM1 dataset, that is, no normalization and no F-score are calculated before the prediction process (Figure 4.2). This is to analyze the dataset without any preprocessing so that we can observe the difference when SVM is directly implemented.
- **Case 2: No Normalization-Has F-Score:** Here the SVM is applied on the pre-processed JM1 dataset, that is, no normalization is done but F-score is calculated for each metric before the prediction process as shown in Figure 4.3. Thus, we can observe what difference it will make when SVM is applied to F-Scored sequence data.
- **Case 3: Has Normalization-No F-Score:** Here the SVM is also applied to the pre-processed JM1 dataset, that is, normalization is done but no F-score is calculated before the prediction process as shown in Figure 4.4. Thus, we can observe what difference it will make when SVM is directly implemented on normalized data.
- **Case 4: Has Normalization-Has F-Score:** This is an important case because herein the data normalization and F-score is done before applying SVM as shown in Figure 4.5. We can observe what difference it will make when SVM is directly implemented.

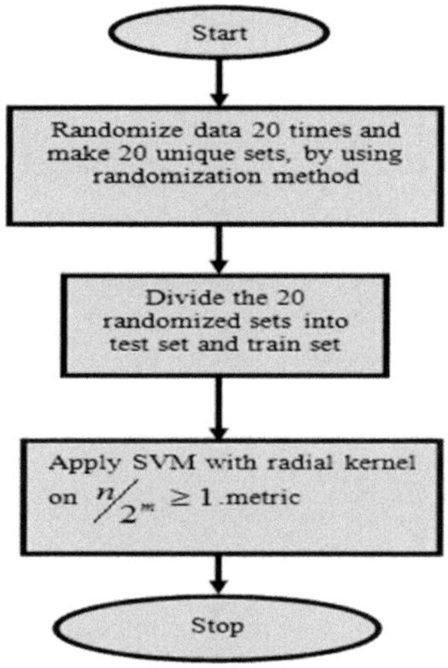

FIGURE 4.2 No normalization-no F-score.

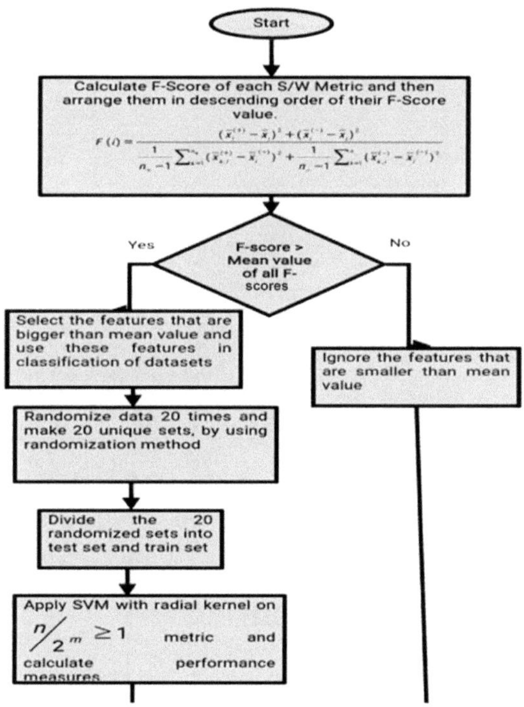

FIGURE 4.3 No normalization-has F-score.

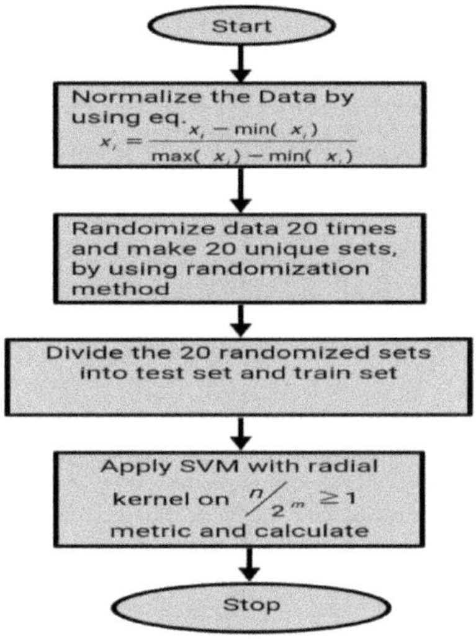

FIGURE 4.4 Has normalization-no F-score.

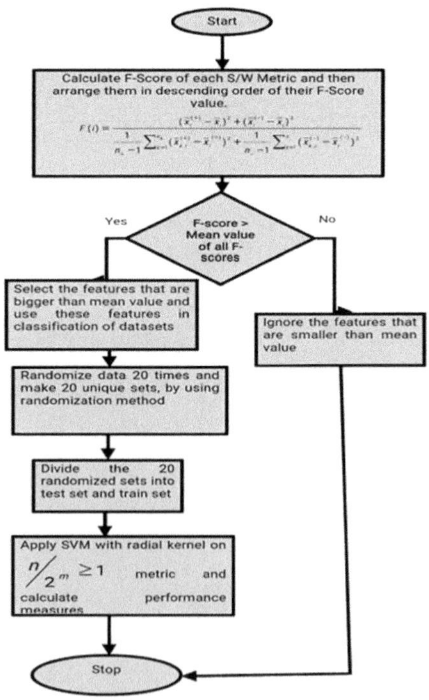

FIGURE 4.5 Has normalization-has F-score.

4.3.3 EVALUATION AND EXPERIMENTAL ENVIRONMENT

The SVM bundle in MATLAB is known as the check and validation sets which are given after to the channels in which facts input into this system at the time of execution. Proper kernel parameters are also defined within the code; here, the default kernel is Gaussian. This gadget includes training that includes of 3107 techniques, with 50 K strains of code. The JM1 dataset provides both magnificence-stage and technique-degree static metrics. At the technique stage, 21 software program product metrics based totally on the product's complexity, size, and vocabulary are given. Five styles of defects such as the wide variety of defects and density of defects are also given. At the magnificence level, values of 10 metrics are computed together with seven metrics. These seven item-orientated (OO) metrics [9] are taken (see Table 4.1) for analyses.

4.3.4 CROSS-VALIDATION

In this chapter, the general tool is records, which presents an attractive guiding principle. First, in addition, the data set is partitioned disjoint subsets: *estimation subset*, used to select the version; and *validation subset*, used to check or validate the version. The motivation here is to validate the version on a one of a kind dataset from that used for parameter estimation. In this manner, we may also use the schooling set to evaluate the performance of diverse candidate fashions, and thereby chooses the "pleasant" one. There is, however, a wonderful possibility that the version with appearing parameter values so selected may additionally turn out to be overfitting the validation subset. To protect towards the opportunity, the generalization performance of the chosen model is measured on the test set, which isn't the same as the validation subset [15].

The technique to move-validation described is called the holdout method. There are different editions of go-validation that find their very own uses in exercise, especially while there may be an absence of labeled examples. In such state of affairs, we may use multifold pass-validation by using dividing the set of N examples into K subsets, $K > 1$; this assumes that K is divisible into N. The model is educated on all of the subsets besides for one, and the validation mistakes are measured by means of testing it on the subset omitted. This system is repeated for a total of okay trials, whenever the usage of an exceptional subset for validation. The performance of the model is assessed by using averaging the squared mistakes underneath validation: it may require too much computation for the reason that version has to be trained ok times, where $1 < K \leq N$. When the quantity of labeled examples, N, is severely restrained, we may use the extreme form of multifold pass-validation referred to as the go away-one-out method. In this situation, N–1 examples are used to educate the model, and the version is proven by means of checking out it on instance omitted. The test is repeated for a total of N times, whenever leaving out a one of a kind instance for validation. The squared errors under validation are then averaged over the N trials of the test [15].

4.3.5 ACCURACY EVALUATION

1. **Accuracy:** It is also referred to as an accurate class rate. It is defined as the ratio of the number of modules correctly expected to the full number of modules [3]:

$$\text{Accuracy} = (\text{TP} + \text{TN})/\text{TP} + \text{TN} + \text{FP} + \text{FN}$$

2. **Precision:** It is likewise known as correctness. It is defined because the ratio of the quantity of modules is effectively anticipated as defective to the whole quantity of modules predicted as faulty. It is calculated as follows [26]:

$$\text{Precision} = \text{TP}/\text{TP} + \text{FP}$$

3. **Recall:** It is likewise called disorder detection fee. It is defined because the ratio of the number of modules effectively predicted as faulty to the full number of modules which might be clearly defective. It is calculated as follows:

$$\text{Recall} = \text{TP}/\text{TP} + \text{FN}$$

Both precision and consideration are essential overall performance measures. The better the precision, the much less effort wasted in trying out and inspection; and the better don't forget, the less defective modules go undetected. However, there's an exchange off between precision and recollect [42]. For example, if a model predicts only one module as defective and this module is truly faulty, the model's precision might be one. However, the versions do not forget might be low if there are other faulty modules. As every other instance, if a model predicts all modules as defective, its consider might be one but its precision may be low. Therefore, F-measure is needed which combines take into account and precision in an unmarried efficiency degree.

$$\text{F-measure} = (2 \times \text{Precision} \times \text{Recall})/\text{Precision} + \text{Recall}$$

4.4 RESULTS AND DISCUSSIONS

➤ **Case: 1 No Normalization-No F-Score:** Table 4.5 shows the results of using SVM with the No Normalization-No F-Score strategy for twenty OO metrics (or the original SVM algorithm). When both normalization and F-Score are not done, the accuracy is only 79% and it is increasing when the number of metrics decreases. Hence, by using some techniques we can improve the prediction efficiency of the SVM.

TABLE 4.5 Results of No Normalization-No F-Score

TN	FN	FP	TP	Accuracy	Precision
2410	503	168	117	0.790181	0.410526
2416	487	183	112	0.790494	0.379661
2448	485	174	91	0.793934	0.343396
2407	525	162	104	0.785178	0.390977
2438	486	170	104	0.794872	0.379562
2391	508	193	106	0.780801	0.354515
2384	525	180	109	0.77955	0.377163
2407	548	144	99	0.783615	0.407407
2440	488	162	108	0.796748	0.4
2388	529	171	110	0.781113	0.391459
2382	518	191	107	0.778299	0.35906
2396	531	171	100	0.780488	0.369004
2417	517	158	106	0.788931	0.401515
2391	521	173	113	0.782989	0.395105
2430	500	157	111	0.794559	0.414179
2401	535	168	94	0.780175	0.358779
2401	494	176	127	0.790494	0.419142
2426	489	163	120	0.796123	0.424028
2412	494	172	120	0.791745	0.410959
2406	474	207	111	0.787054	0.349057

➢ **Case 2: No Normalization-Has F-Score:** Table 4.6 shows the results of No Normalization-Has F-Score for twenty-one OO Metrics. It is realized that in some cases, the accuracy reaches to more than 80%. Clearly, using SVM with F-score improves the accuracy of prediction.

TABLE 4.6 Results of No Normalization-Has F-Score

TN	FN	FP	TP	Accuracy	Precision
2391	510	175	122	0.785804	41.07744
2402	506	167	123	0.789556	42.41379
2391	502	186	119	0.784866	39.01639
2415	480	180	123	0.793621	40.59406
2524	328	48	298	**0.882427**	86.12717
2433	479	180	106	0.793934	37.06294
2449	482	156	111	**0.8005**	41.57303
2384	514	181	119	0.782677	39.66667
2398	502	171	127	0.789556	42.61745
2419	505	172	102	0.788305	37.22628
2385	522	173	118	0.782677	40.54983
2385	508	188	117	0.782364	38.36066
8584	1073	193	1030	**0.88364**	84.21913
2417	517	159	105	0.788618	39.77273
240	506	178	114	0.786116	39.0411
2385	532	155	126	0.785178	44.83986
2394	490	202	112	0.783615	35.66879
2422	484	171	121	0.795184	41.43836
2391	500	195	112	0.782677	36.48208
2410	530	146	112	0.788618	43.41085

(Bold values are greater than 80%).

➢ **Case 3: Has Normalization-No F-Score:** Table 4.7 shows the results of Has Normalization-No F-Score strategy for twenty OO Metrics. It is clearly recognized that using Normalization in SVM achieves more number of best results (i.e., accuracies are greater than 80%).

TABLE 4.7 Results of Has Normalization-No F-Score

TN	FN	FP	TP	Accuracy	Precision
2400	532	152	115	0.786183	0.430712
2400	497	186	115	0.786429	0.38206
2388	538	175	97	0.777048	0.356618
2392	499	184	122	0.786362	0.398693
2506	328	70	294	**0.875547**	0.807692
2382	487	202	127	0.784553	0.386018
2405	497	179	117	0.788618	0.39527
2375	510	196	117	0.779237	0.373802
2423	522	150	103	0.789556	0.407115
2435	494	161	108	**0.886492**	0.401487
2422	502	171	103	**0.803315**	0.37912
2524	304	59	311	**0.886492**	0.840541
2462	479	150	107	**0.803315**	0.416348
2404	521	164	109	0.785804	0.399267
2513	327	54	304	**0.880863**	0.849162
2418	510	169	101	0.78768	0.374074
2379	518	192	0.9	0.777986	0.362
2411	544	149	94	0.783302	0.386831
2410	514	150	124	0.79237	0.452555
2428	492	163	115	0.795184	0.413669

(Bold values are greater than 80%).

- **Case 4: Has Normalization-Has F-Score:** Table 4.8 shows the results of Has Normalization-Has F-Score strategy with twenty OO Metrics. It is amazing that the number of accuracies greater than 80% is only 2. The combination of both normalization and F-score is not as good as the Has Normalization-No F-Score strategy.

Table 4.9 indicates the general accuracy and precision of every strategy for a given number of metrics. The accuracy of fashions predicted is somewhat optimistic given that they are implemented to the equal dataset from which they are derived. Herein, the first-class variety of metrics is 5 [i.e., LOC, Program Level (L), Branch Count (BR), and Unique Operands] with the No Normalization-Has F-Score method. The graphical representation of this table is shown in Figure 4.6.

TABLE 4.8 Results of Has Normalization-Has F-Score

TN	FN	FP	TP	Accuracy	Precision
2417	509	159	114	0.791185	0.417582
2426	470	182	120	0.796123	0.397351
2421	520	146	111	0.791745	0.431907
2387	526	177	108	0.780175	0.378947
2404	499	190	105	0.784553	0.355932
2428	499	153	123	0.796441	0.445652
2385	536	168	109	0.779862	0.393502
2443	451	176	128	**0.80394**	0.421053
2391	495	202	110	0.782051	0.352564
2416	497	182	103	0.78768	0.361404
2445	480	162	111	0.79925	0.406593
2401	499	184	114	0.786429	0.38255
2375	504	198	121	0.780488	0.37931
2424	485	161	128	0.797999	0.442907
2383	520	190	105	0.777986	0.355932
2401	490	184	123	0.789243	0.400651
2363	533	184	118	0.775797	0.390728
2407	495	178	118	0.789556	0.398649
2431	519	157	91	0.788618	0.366935
2443	468	171	116	**0.800188**	0.404181

(Bold values are greater than 80%).

We also achieved a significance test among the prediction overall performance of SVM and people of the alternative eight as compared models: KNN, Adaboost, bootstrap aggregation techniques (bagging), gradient boosted decision trees (GB), random forests (RF), extremely randomized trees (Trees), and one-class SVMs (one-class) obtained from JM1 dataset (Figure 4.7).

In Figure 4.7, the results offer the numbers of Yes(+), No(+), No(), and Yes() for each performance measure. In brief, it may be determined that SVM significantly outperforms four out of the eight as compared models inaccuracy, that is, there are four Yes(+). It also can be found that SVM is extensively outperformed by using models in precision. However, it achieves drastically higher recall than almost all the different fashions. As

TABLE 4.9 Results of All Strategies by Various Numbers of OO Metrics

No. of OO Metrics	No Normalization, No F-Score				No Normalization, Has F-Score				Has Normalization, No F-Score				Has Normalization, Has F-Score			
	21	**11**	**5**	**2**	**21**	**11**	**5**	**2**	**21**	**11**	**5**	**2**	**21**	**11**	**5**	**2**
Accuracy	78.7	80.2	80.5	**81.1**	79.7	**81.1**	**81.4**	80.9	**80.2**	80.6	80.9	**81.1**	78.9	80.6	81.1	**81.1**
Precision	38.7	46.3	49.7	55.4	44.6	53.1	58.5	55.0	46.0	49.8	54.0	58.1	39.4	48.1	53.8	55.8

(Bold values imply the best for a given number of metrics).

defined earlier, there is a change-off between precision and don't forget, however, the F-degree considers their harmonic imply that takes both of them similarly into account. It can be observed that SVM achieves better F-measure than all the compared models. This seems to suggest that, with none know-how of the distribution of facts, the quality measures to be used are accuracy and precision that permit locating problems with classifiers. In summary, the No Normalization-Has F-Score method achieves the very best accuracy (81.43%). SVM achieves higher F-measure than five of the eight as compared fashions. There is no any significant difference between SVM and all fashions in F-measure.

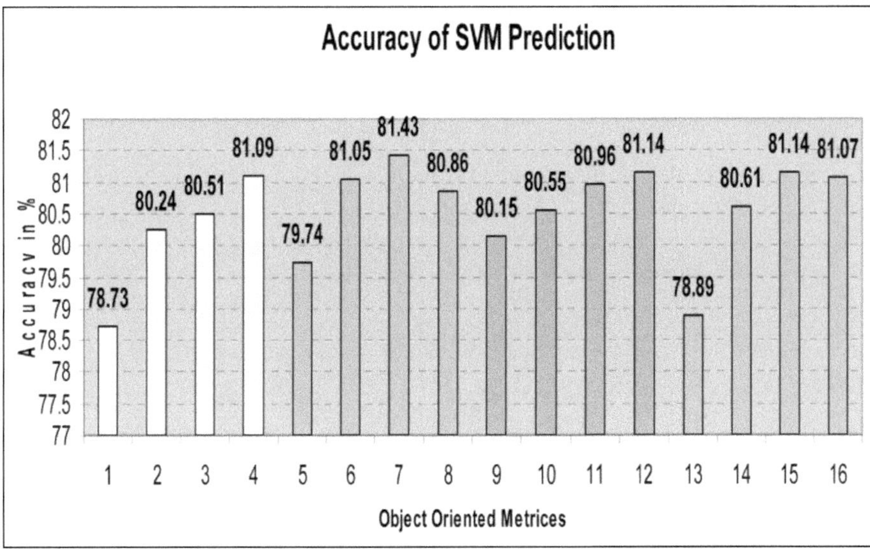

FIGURE 4.6 Accuracy of SVM prediction.

4.5 CONCLUSIONS

Software exceptional guarantee procedure specializes in the identification and removal of faults quickly from the artifacts which can be generated and ultimately used in the improvement of software program. Software fault prediction is one of the strategies, which might be performed rapturously all through the very early stage of the software program development lifestyle cycle. Fault prediction statistics no longer only factors to the want for improved excellence throughout the improvement, however, additionally presents statistics to recognize suitable verification and validation activities on the way to improve the effectiveness. The effectiveness of a fault-prediction technique is verified by using teaching it over a part of a few acknowledged fault data and measuring its performance towards the other a part of the fault facts.

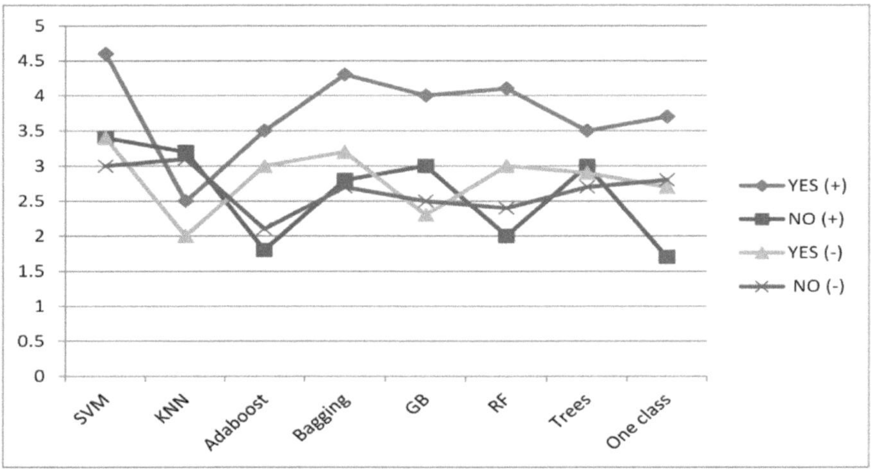

FIGURE 4.7 Prediction performance of SVM and other machine learning methods.

This bankruptcy proposed a new method combining SVM and characteristic selection incorporating with various procedures between records normalization and F-score; that is, No Normalization-No F-Score, No Normalization-Has F-Score, Has Normalization-No F-Score, and Has Normalization-Has F-Score. It has been determined that the accuracy and precision of SVM are biggest with the No Normalization-Has F-Score technique, that is, 81.43% in the case of the use of five item-oriented metrics namely LOC, program level (L), branch count (BR), and unique operands. Hence, the above metrics have significant susceptible in defect prone modules. On the alternative hand, normalizing the statistics is not powerful due to larger accuracy and precision than the different three strategies.

From the acquired outcomes, it became located that there has been no single approach that would provide the fine consequences in all instances. However, for specific vital programs, wherein ignoring faults may be vital, the usage of fault prediction might not be effective if it has high FNs. Thus, in addition, works can be finished on accomplishing extra empirical studies with other varieties of datasets with embedded four strategies.

KEYWORDS

- **branch count**
- **false negative**
- **false positive**
- **gradient boosted**
- **machine learning**
- **metrics data program**

REFERENCES

1. Afzal, U., Mahmood, T., & Shaikh, Z., (2016). Intelligent software product line configurations: A literature review. *Computer Standards and Interfaces*, *48*, 30–48.
2. Akour, M., Alsmadi, I., & Alazzam, I., (2017). Software fault proneness prediction: A comparative study between bagging, boosting, and stacking ensemble and base learner methods. *International Journal of Data Analysis Techniques and Strategies*, *9*(1), 1–16.
3. Alexandridis, A., Chondrodima, E., & Sarimveis, H., (2016). Cooperative learning for radial basis function networks using particle swarm optimization. *Applied Soft Computing*, *49*, 485–497.
4. Alsmadi, I., & Najadat, H., (2011). Evaluating the change of software fault behavior with dataset attributes based on categorical correlation. *Advances in Engineering Software*, *42*(8), 535–546.
5. Arar, Ö. F., & Ayan, K., (2016). Deriving thresholds of software metrics to predict faults on open source software: Replicated case studies. *Expert Systems with Applications*, *61*, 106–121.
6. Arisholm, E., Briand, L. C., & Fuglerud, M., (2007). Data mining techniques for building fault-proneness models in telecom java software. *18th IEEE International Symposium on Software Reliability (ISSRE'07)* (pp. 215–224).

7. Basili, V., McGarry, F., Pajerski, R., & Zelkowitz, M., (2002). Lessons learned from 25 years of process improvement: The rise and fall of the NASA software engineering laboratory. *Proceedings of the IEEE and ACM International Conference on Software Engineering*, 69–79.
8. Catal, C., & Diri, B., (2009). A systematic review of software fault prediction studies. *Expert Systems with Applications*, *36*(4), 7346–7354.
9. Chen, J. S., & Cheng, C. H., (2008). Extracting classification rule of software diagnosis using modified MEPA. *Expert Systems with Applications*, *34*(1), 411–418.
10. Chidamber, S., & Kemerer, C., (1994). A metrics suite for object-oriented design. *IEEE Transactions on Software Engineering, 20*(6), 476–493.
11. Demetgul, M., Unal, M., Tansel, I. N., & Yazıcıoğlu, O., (2011). Fault diagnosis on bottle filling plant using a genetic-based neural network. *Advances in Engineering Software*, *42*(12), 1051–1058.
12. Durán, A., Benavides, D., Segura, S., Trinidad, P., & Ruiz-Cortés, A., (2015). FLAME: A formal framework for the automated analysis of software product lines validated by automated specification testing. *Software and Systems Modeling*, 1–34.
13. Elish, K. O., & Elish, M. O., (2008). Predicting defect-prone software modules using support vector machines. *Journal of Systems and Software*, *81*(5), 649–660.
14. Elish, M. O., Al-Yafei, A. H., & Al-Mulhem, M., (2011). Empirical comparison of three metrics suites for fault prediction in packages of object-oriented systems: A case study of Eclipse. *Advances in Engineering Software*, *42*(10), 852–859.
15. Gondra, I., (2008). Applying machine learning to software fault-proneness prediction. *Journal of Systems and Software*, *81*(2), 186–195.
16. Goyal, R., Chandra, P., & Singh, Y., (2016). A review of metrics and modeling techniques in software fault prediction model development. *Covenant Journal of Informatics and Communication Technology*, *3*(2), 23–51.
17. Grbac, T. G., & Huljenić, D., (2015). On the probability distribution of faults in complex software systems. *Information and Software Technology*, *58*, 250–258.
18. Gu, S., Cheng, R., & Jin, Y., (2016). Feature selection for high-dimensional classification using a competitive swarm optimizer. *Soft Computing*, 1–12.
19. Guo, L., Ma, Y., Cukic, B., & Singh, H., (2004). Robust prediction of fault-proneness by random forests. In: *15th IEEE International Symposium on Software Reliability Engineering (ISSRE 2004)* (pp. 417–428).
20. Hamill, M., & Goseva-Popstojanova, K., (2017). Analyzing and predicting effort associated with finding and fixing software faults. *Information and Software Technology*, *87*, 1–18.
21. Heinrich, R., Merkle, P., Henss, J., & Paech, B., (2017). Integrating business process simulation and information system simulation for performance prediction. *Software and Systems Modeling*, *16*(1), 257–277.
22. Immonen, A., & Niemelä, E., (2008). Survey of reliability and availability prediction methods from the viewpoint of software architecture. *Software and Systems Modeling*, *7*(1), 49–65.
23. Ivanciuc, O., (2007). Applications of support vector machines in chemistry. *Reviews in Computational Chemistry*, *23*, 291.

24. Kapila, H., Kaur, D., & Majithia, S., (2016). A review on software fault prediction technique using different dataset. *International Journal of Technology and Computing, 2*(5).
25. Karimian, F., & Babamir, S. M., (2016). Evaluation of classifiers in software fault-proneness prediction. *Journal of AI and Data Mining.*
26. Keerthi, S. S., & Lin, C. J., (2003). Asymptotic behaviors of support vector machines with Gaussian kernel. *Neural Computation, 15*(7), 1667–1689.
27. Koru, A., & Tian, J., (2003). An empirical comparison and characterization of high defect and high complexity modules. *Journal of Systems and Software, 67*, 153–163.
28. Kumar, L., Misra, S., & Rath, S. K., (2017). An empirical analysis of the effectiveness of software metrics and fault prediction model for identifying faulty classes. *Computer Standards and Interfaces, 53*, 1–32.
29. Kumar, R., & Duraisamy, S., (2016). Fault prediction in object oriented systems using adaptive neuro-fuzzy inference system model. *Asian Journal of Research in Social Sciences and Humanities, 6*(12), 944–950.
30. Lahsasna, A., & Seng, W. C., (2017). An improved genetic-fuzzy system for classification and data analysis. *Expert Systems with Applications, 83*(15), 49–62.
31. Lee, S. Y., Li, D., & Li, Y., (2016). An investigation of essential topics on software fault-proneness prediction. *IEEE International Symposium on System and Software Reliability (ISSSR),* 37–46.
32. Li, W., Huang, Z., & Li, Q., (2016). Three-way decisions based software defect prediction. *Knowledge-Based Systems, 91*, 263–274.
33. LI, Y., Bai, B. D., & Jiao, L. C., (2001). The mechanism of classification for support vector machines. *Systems Engineering and Electronics, 23*(9), 25–27.
34. Liu, W., Liu, S., Gu, Q., Chen, J., Chen, X., & Chen, D., (2016). Empirical studies of a two-stage data preprocessing approach for software fault prediction. *IEEE Transactions on Reliability, 65*(1), 38–53.
35. Ma, W., Chen, L., Yang, Y., Zhou, Y., & Xu, B., (2016). Empirical analysis of network measures for effort-aware fault-proneness prediction. *Information and Software Technology, 69*, 50–70.
36. Mair, C., Kadoda, G., Leflel, M., Phapl, L., Schofield, K., Shepperd, M., & Webster, S., (2000). An investigation of machine learning-based prediction systems. *Journal of Systems and Software, 53*(1), 23–29.
37. Morfidis, K., & Kostinakis, K., (2017). Seismic parameters' combinations for the optimum prediction of the damage state of R/C buildings using neural networks. *Advances in Engineering Software, 106*, 1–16.
38. Pendharkar, P. C., (2010). Exhaustive and heuristic search approaches for learning a software defect prediction model. *Engineering Applications of Artificial Intelligence, 23*(1), 34–40.
39. Rathore, S. S., & Kumar, S., (2017). Linear and non-linear heterogeneous ensemble methods to predict the number of faults in software systems. *Knowledge-Based Systems, 119*, 232–256.
40. Rizvi, S. W. A., Singh, V. K., & Khan, R. A., (2016). The state of the art in software reliability prediction: Software metrics and fuzzy logic perspective. In: *Information Systems Design and Intelligent Applications* (pp. 629–637). Springer India.

41. Singh, P., Pal, N. R., Verma, S., & Vyas, O. P., (2016). Fuzzy rule-based approach for software fault prediction. *IEEE Transactions on Systems, Man, and Cybernetics: Systems*, *47*(5), 826–837.
42. Szvetits, M., & Zdun, U., (2016). Systematic literature review of the objectives, techniques, kinds, and architectures of models at runtime. *Software and Systems Modeling*, *15*(1), 31–69.
43. Visentini, I., Snidaro, L., & Foresti, G. L., (2016). Diversity-aware classifier ensemble selection via f-score. *Information Fusion*, *28*, 24–43.
44. Witten, I., & Frank, E., (2005). *Data Mining: Practical Machine Learning Tools and Techniques* (2nd edn.). Morgan Kaufmann, San Francisco.
45. Wulf, D., & Bertschn, V., (2017). A natural language generation approach to support understanding and traceability of multi-dimensional preferential sensitivity analysis in multi-criteria decision making. *Expert Systems with Applications*, *83*(15), 131–144.
46. Xiao, Q., (2017). Recurrent neural network system using probability graph model optimization. *Applied Intelligence*, *46*(4), 889–897.
47. Xu, T., Gondra, I., & Chiu, D. K., (2017). A maximum partial entropy-based method for multiple-instance concept learning. *Applied Intelligence*, *46*(4), 865–875.
48. Yadav, H. B., & Yadav, D. K., (2015). A fuzzy logic-based approach for phase-wise software defects prediction using software metrics. *Information and Software Technology*, *63*, 44–57.
49. Yang, Y., Harman, M., Krinke, J., Islam, S., Binkley, D., Zhou, Y., & Xu, B., (2016). An empirical study on dependence clusters for effort-aware fault-proneness prediction. In: *2016 31st IEEE/ACM International Conference on Automated Software Engineering (ASE)* (pp. 296–307).
50. Zhang, W., Yang, Y., & Wang, Q., (2015). Using Bayesian regression and EM algorithm with missing handling for software effort prediction. *Information and Software Technology*, *58*, 58–70.
51. Zhao, Y., Yang, Y., Lu, H., Liu, J., Leung, H., Wu, Y., & Xu, B., (2016). Understanding the value of considering client usage context in package cohesion for fault-proneness prediction. *Automated Software Engineering*, 1–61.
52. Zhao, Y., Yang, Y., Lu, H., Zhou, Y., Song, Q., & Xu, B., (2015). An empirical analysis of package-modularization metrics: Implications for software fault-proneness. *Information and Software Technology*, *57*, 186–203.

CHAPTER 5

Antennas for Biomedical Applications Using RF Energy Harvesting

NEETA SINGH,[1] SACHIN KUMAR,[2] and BINOD KUMAR KANAUJIA[3]

[1]*Ambedkar Institute of Advanced Communication Technologies and Research, Delhi–110031, India, E-mail: neeta.singh90@gmail.com*

[2]*School of Electronics Engineering, Kyungpook National University, Daegu–41566, Republic of Korea, E-mail: gupta.sachin0708@gmail.com*

[3]*School of Computational and Integrative Sciences, Jawaharlal Nehru University, New Delhi–110067, India, E-mail: bkkanaujia@ieee.org*

ABSTRACT

The demand for wireless power transmission is increasing day-by-day to power up smart sensing and low energy devices. The most emerging field in the environment of wireless power transmission is a health monitoring system, which is power-driven by RF energy harvesting. RF energy harvesting is accomplished by using a device called "rectenna." The rectenna consists of a sensing antenna that receives ambient signals available freely in the environment and sends them to the rectifier, which converts the received AC signal into the DC waveform. Further, the converted DC voltage can be used in biomedical devices for health monitoring. This device may be implanted or wearable depending upon the requirements and it ensures monitoring of different organs of the body remotely. Due to the use of RF energy harvesting, the often replacement of device battery is not required and a device can monitor health for the long term or sometimes everlasting. The design and analysis of different antenna types used for RF energy harvesting and different techniques involved in the smart health monitoring system are reviewed and presented in this chapter. The chapter also investigates the advantages of printed rectenna such as light-weight, compact size, and their compatibility with the body organs.

5.1 INTRODUCTION

The internet of things (IoT) devices show rapid development in various fields such as smart agriculture, smart cities, smart communication, and smart healthcare. Nowadays, healthcare becomes an essential part of life especially for aging people [1], and by using IoT the patient information can be changed from physical phenomenon to digital signals. The IoT devices communicate with each other and share information of the patient directly, which helps a doctor in the prescription of medication [2]. Figure 5.1 shows a block diagram of the wireless monitoring system.

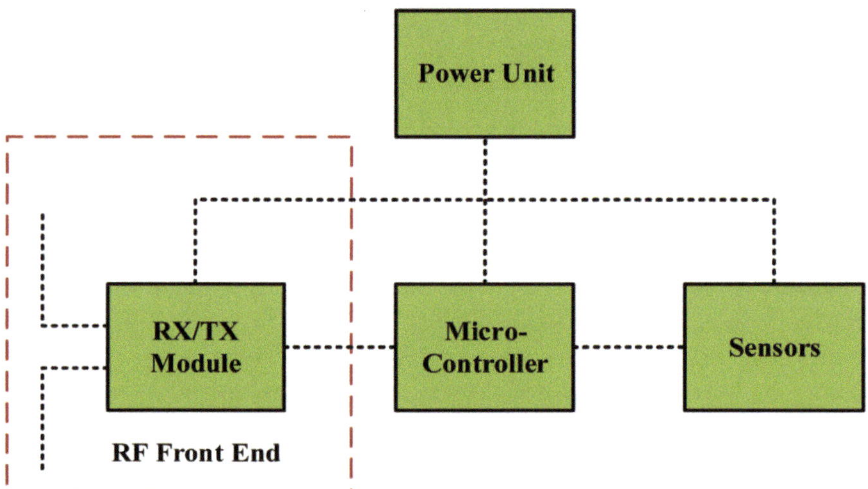

FIGURE 5.1 Wireless monitoring system.

To implement such technology, devices that can provide a regular power to the system or wireless battery is required, which does not necessitate replacement of the battery. The objectives of wireless power technology can be fulfilled by a device called "rectenna." Rectenna is a wireless battery consisting of a receiving antenna and rectifier circuit [3] and provides a continuous power supply to the connected device/system [4]. The receiving antenna collects the freely available RF signals from the environment and converts them into useful DC power with the help of a rectifier. The sensing antenna can be of any types: horn antenna [5], dipole antenna [6], monopole antenna [7], Yagi-Uda antenna [8], microstrip patch antenna [9, 10], and spiral antenna [11]. A circularly polarized (CP) antenna may be used for obtaining high-efficiency wireless power transfer. The most commonly used antennas that show circular polarization are the helical antenna, spiral antenna, truncated microstrip antenna, square, and circular patch antenna with loaded slits/slots.

The sensing antennas must be of the same polarization as transmitting devices to avoid polarization mismatch. If the polarization mismatch between the transmitting and receiving signals increases, the received power gets affected. The power received will be zero if both the signals are orthogonal to each other. Hence, if the receiving antenna is linearly polarized, then the transmitting antenna must also have linear polarization, and if the signal orientation changes due to some obstacles, the power loss will be high. To increase RF to DC conversion efficiency, the circular polarized antennas are preferred, as they receive signals with high efficiency irrespective of the change of direction or angle of the signal [12, 13]. Early research in the field of wireless power transmission was conducted by N. Tesla, in early 1890 on a magnetic coil [14]. But his experiments were failed and do not show the benefits of the device. Then, in 1960, W. C. Brown introduces a device called rectenna that consists of a sensing antenna and rectifier. He tested his research on a helicopter, which worked on 2.45 GHz.

5.2 DIFFERENT WAYS TO INVESTIGATE THE HEALTH

Nowadays smart healthcare is an essential part of day-to-day life. The sensing device used to investigate the patient's health may be an implantable antenna, wearable antenna, or the sensors connected with the internet. By using a bio-telemetry system, the doctors can analyze the medical need and give correct medication to the patients. This technique helps the doctor to connect all the time with the patient and monitor their health regularly.

5.2.1 WEARABLE ANTENNA/SENSORS

Recently, various researchers are working on healthcare systems that use telemedicine technology, which increases life expectancy and reduces the effective cost for medication. The non-invasive wearable sensors provide painless access to the human body [15]. Figure 5.2 illustrates a block diagram of the wearable system.

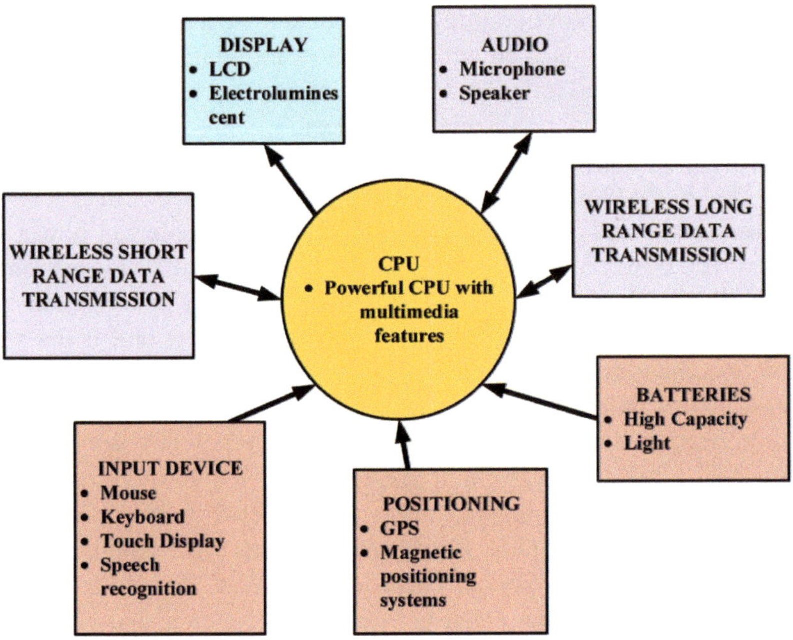

FIGURE 5.2 Block diagram of the wearable system.

The wearable sensors consist of wearable antennas, which are placed on the body to measure the anomalies in the patient body and transmit information to the monitoring platform with the help of IoT as shown in Figure 5.3. The wearable antenna is fabricated on fabric-based material or knitted on the patient's clothes and gives better sensitivity than the printed sensors. This section focuses on the types and fabrication of wearable antennas. These types of antennas are roughly categorized into two groups which are discussed in the following subsections.

5.2.1.1 CONVENTIONAL WEARABLE DESIGNS

The conventional wearable antennas are commonly used for biomedical applications including microstrip patch, dipole, folded dipole, printed spiral, and planar inverted-F antenna (PIFA) [16]. These antennas are commonly used due to their low cost and easy fabrication. As microstrip patch antennas are compact in size and easily manufactured, they are most often used.

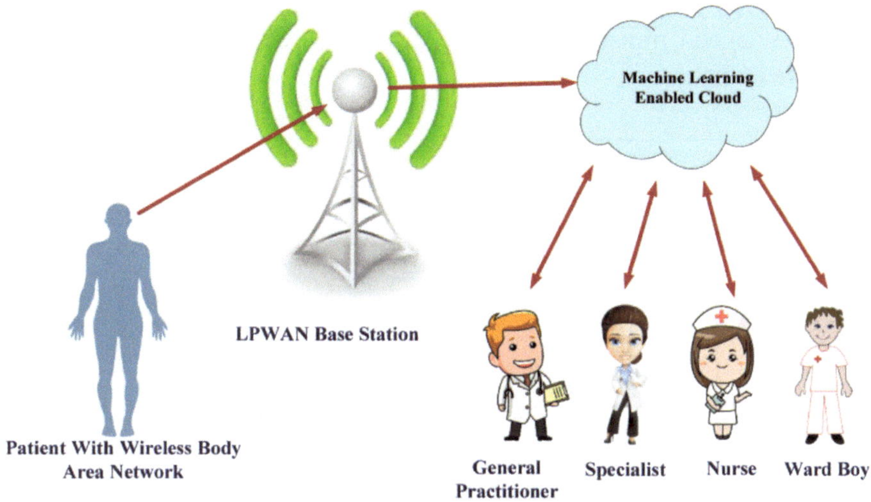

FIGURE 5.3 Layout of the healthcare monitoring system.

The EM waves can penetrated and absorbed by the human body; sometimes these radiations are very much dangerous and can cause serious health issues. For wearable antennas, a low value of specific absorption rate (SAR) is needed that does not affect the human body. The microstrip patch antenna has a higher SAR because of minor lobe radiations. The SAR can be reduced by the following methods:

1. The feed position of the antenna should be carefully chosen so that most of the radiations are in the major lobe.
2. A reflector or EM wave absorber can be used that can reflect/absorb the back radiations.
3. The ground plane should be a perfect conductor that radiates all the waves in a forward direction.

These sensors are embedded in wearable clothes that can easily and continuously monitor the health of the person [17]. Different material and fabrication techniques are used for the development of conventional wearable antennas. In Ref. [18], a novel PIFA antenna comprised of a triangular slot and fleece material substrate was reported; the PIFA shows dual-band response. The fleece material is used due to its easy availability and on-body integration.

In Ref. [19], a wearable flexible PIFA for single and dual-band operation was reported as shown in Figure 5.4. The flexible substrate antenna shows enhanced transmission power as compared to the rigid material substrate antennas.

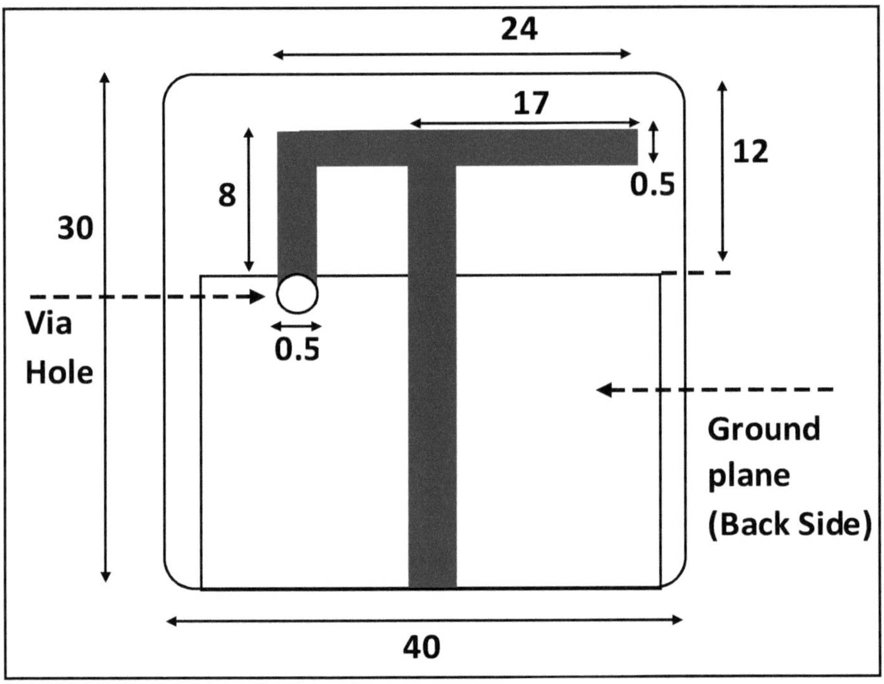

FIGURE 5.4 PIFA design of the antenna (dimensions in mm).

A broadband wearable antenna resonating at the FM band (87.5–108 MHz) was presented in Ref. [20]. The folded dipole multi-frequency antenna design is shown in Figure 5.5.

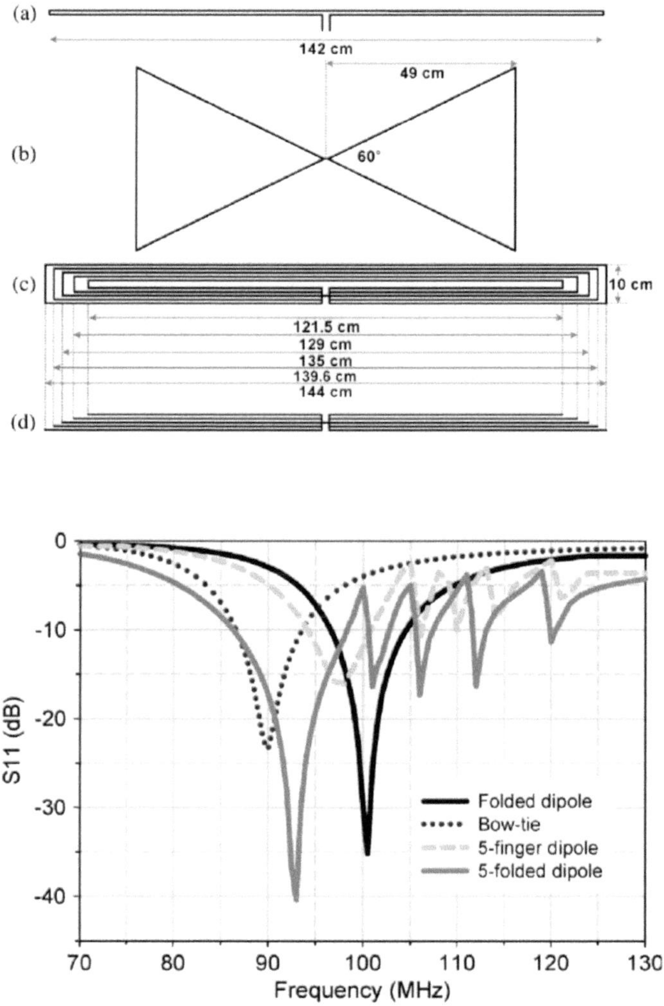

FIGURE 5.5 (a) Folded dipole, (b) bow-tie antenna, (c) 5 finger dipole, (d) 5 folded dipole, (e) reflection coefficients of the antenna [20].

The conventional wearable antennas radiate harmful radiations which penetrate inside the human body through the skin and absorbed by the cells. Body-worn antennas can cause serious health issues; hence, these antennas must be operated into the safe limits. The limits can be determined by means of SAR and the antennas with less SAR are widely used. In recent times, various materials are in existence to suppress SAR.

5.2.2 TEXTILE ANTENNA DESIGNS

The wearable systems have been designed according to the user's situation and work all the time without affecting the user's activities. For wearable and body-worn applications, flexible textile antennas embedded into clothes, blankets, and bedsheets of the patients are used, which continuously monitors the health of the individual.

An ultra-wideband (UWB) textile antenna was reported in Ref. [21]. This antenna uses a flannel fabric textile material substrate with a permittivity of 1.7 that provides 17 GHz bandwidth as shown in Figure 5.6. The thickness of the substrate is 3 mm.

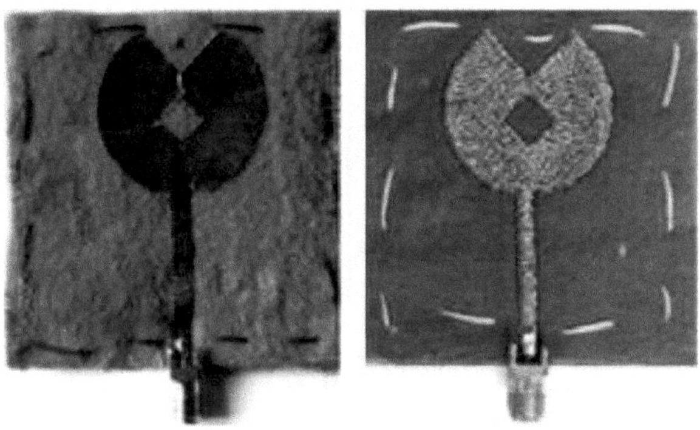
(a) (b)

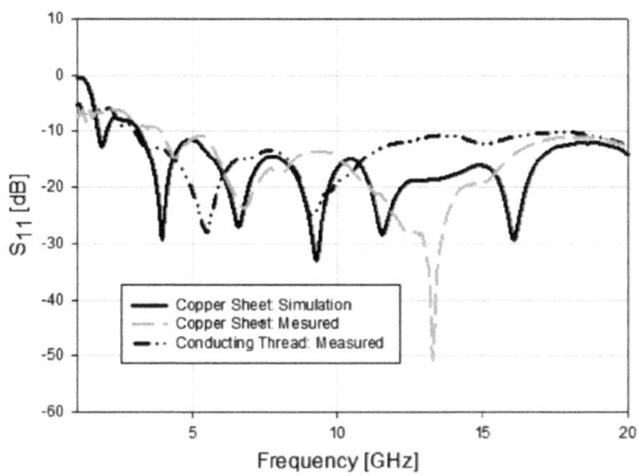

(c)

FIGURE 5.6 UWB antenna (a) front view, (b) back view, (c) reflection coefficients of the antenna [21].

The microstrip feed line textile antenna with circular polarization is needed to avoid polarization mismatch [22]. A wearable CP antenna with truncated corners of the patch is shown in Figure 5.7. This is useful for mobile applications where the patient is not stable and its polarization is changing continuously, the reported antenna radiates efficiently irrespective of its orientation.

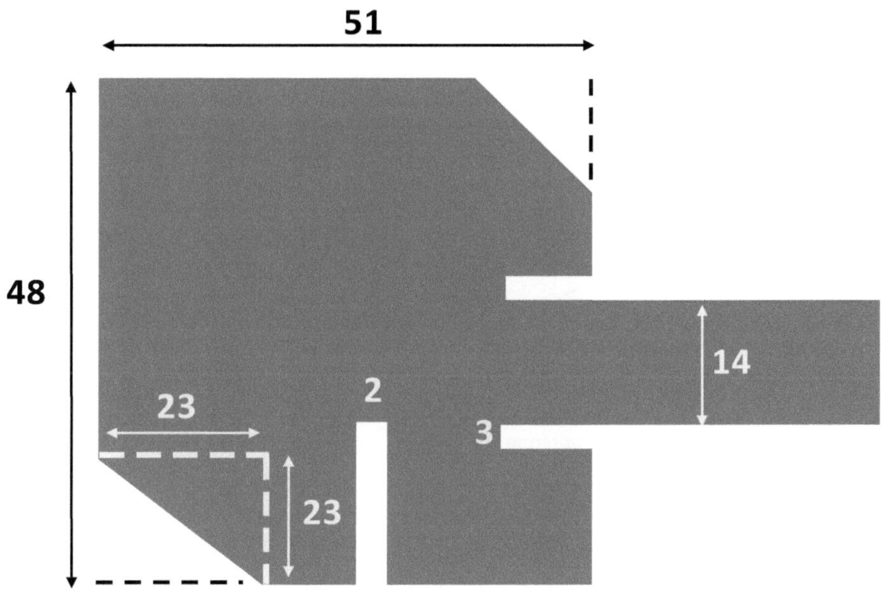

FIGURE 5.7 Circularly polarized antenna (dimensions in mm).

In Ref. [23], a button-shaped wearable Yagi antenna array was presented. The antenna array resonates at 2.45 GHz showing applications for wireless body area networks (WBAN). It is suitable for embedding into clothes due to its robustness, low cost, rigidness, and low profile. The antenna is composed of two PEC layers, one for a ground plane and second for Yagi as shown in Figure 5.8. A thick substrate with relative permittivity of 6.6 is used between the upper and lower layers.

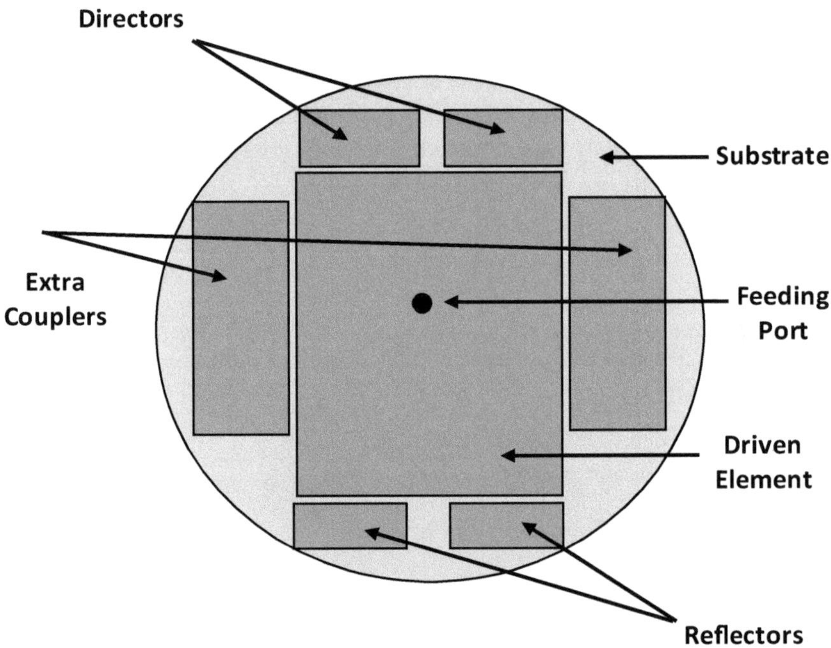

FIGURE 5.8 Layout of Yagi antenna.

A textile microstrip patch antenna with circular polarization and operating at 2.45 GHz was presented in Ref. [24]. The aramid fabric was used for fabricating the reported rectangular ring antenna as shown in Figure 5.9. The circular polarization helps to obtain high-efficiency.

5.2.3 IMPLANTABLE ANTENNAS

The implantable sensor is a source of communication between the external and internal devices which helps in the transmission of information. For biomedical applications, the antenna must be efficient and compact that can match the requirements of the implantable device. Nowadays, implantable antennas are used for sugar level checks, blood pressure measurements, insulin pumps, endoscopy, deep brain stimulation, glucose monitoring, etc. But still, the researchers are facing several challenges related to the implantable device's performance. The miniaturization is a big issue in biomedical antennas; however, the size of the device affects the radiation characteristics of the antenna. Therefore, researches are still going on to achieve good radiation characteristics and compact size. The most important objective of the healthcare system using IoT is to provide an uninterrupted report of the patient to the external base station. The various components used in the wireless implantable system are shown in Figure 5.10.

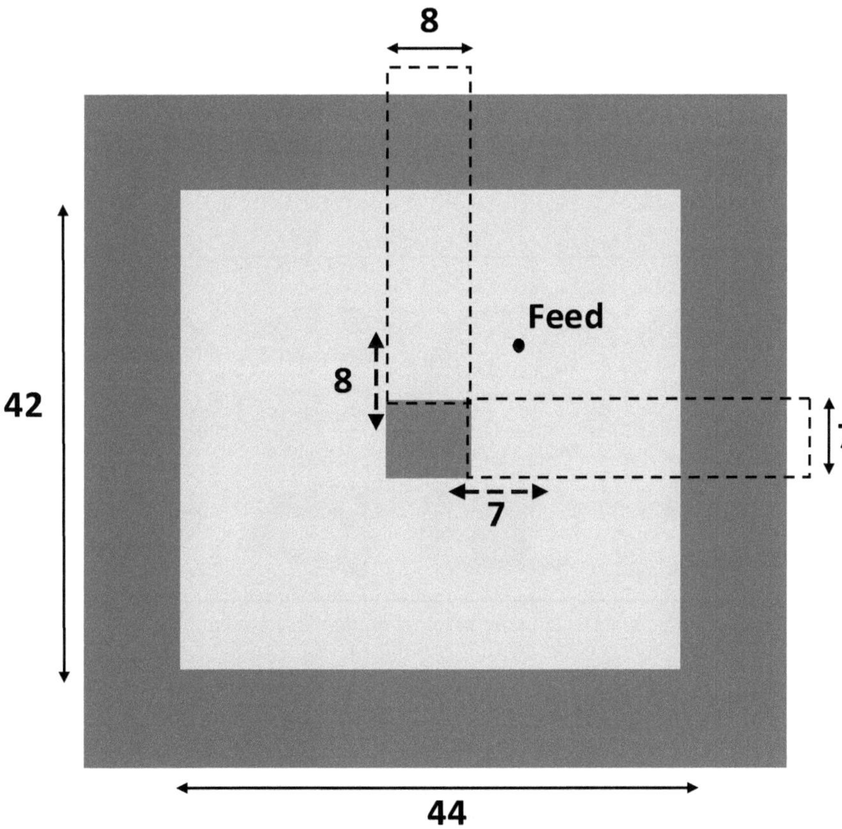

FIGURE 5.9 Circularly polarized antenna with dimensions [24].

5.2.3.1 *INSULATION*

It is a material used in implantable devices to protect the body from the harmful effects of the EM waves. This material can be used in any part of the body. The essential requirement of insulation to work satisfactorily in the environment of the human body is processability, bio-adhesion, bio-compatibility, and bio-functioning.

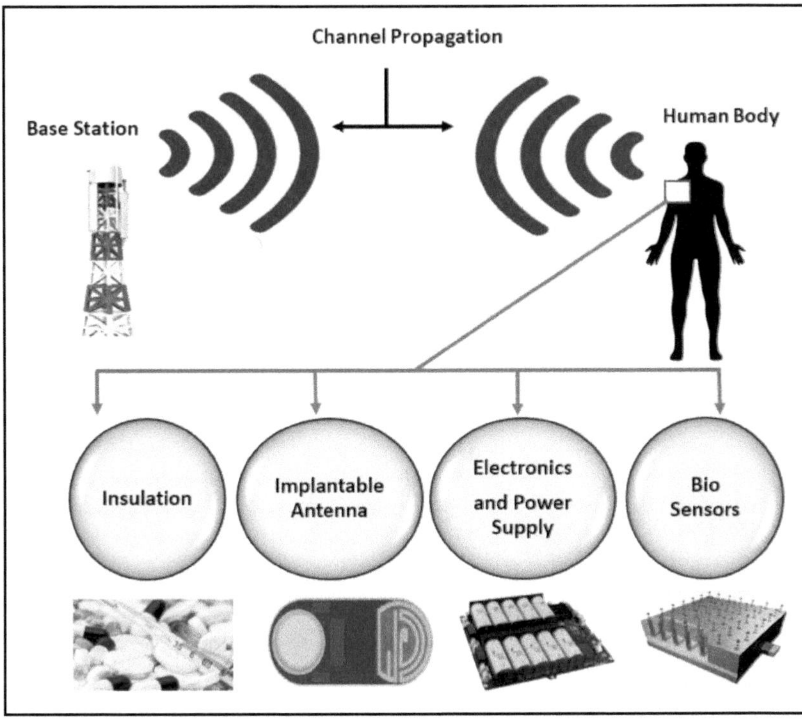

FIGURE 5.10 Components used in the wireless implantable system.

5.2.3.2 IMPLANTABLE ANTENNAS

Without IoT, the base station should be in a few meters range whereas by using IoT, the home monitoring can be done even for long distances. For wireless communication, the radiation efficiency, coupling factor with the body tissues, and miniaturization should be in the specified range.

5.2.3.3 ELECTRONICS AND POWER SUPPLY

The integration of the implantable antenna and various electronic equipment such as micro-controller, transmitter system, CPU, and data communication device are needed for the wireless monitoring system. The wired power supply requires a large space and also affects the lifetime of the equipment. RF energy harvesting provides the best solution to this problem. The rectenna is a device through which RF energy can be harvested and utilized when needed.

5.2.3.4 BIO-SENSORS AND BIO-ACTUATORS

Bio-sensors are the device which works as a transducer to convert bio-signals into the electrical measurable signals that give data report of the patient to the specialists. Various types of sensors such as bacterial sensors, DNA sensors, optical sensors, enzymatic sensors, and surface plasmon resonance sensors have been introduced for bio-medical applications.

The researcher must take care of all environment of the human body to design an implantable antenna for biomedical applications [25]. As shown in Figure 5.11, the surrounding environment of the antenna is divided into multiple layers. The outermost layer represented by 5 is free-space (external environment), layers 4 and 3 are of human tissues which include muscles, fat, and skin. Layer 2 is a biocompatible material used for insulation so that the device will not affect the body tissues. Layer 1 contains air and is called the origin.

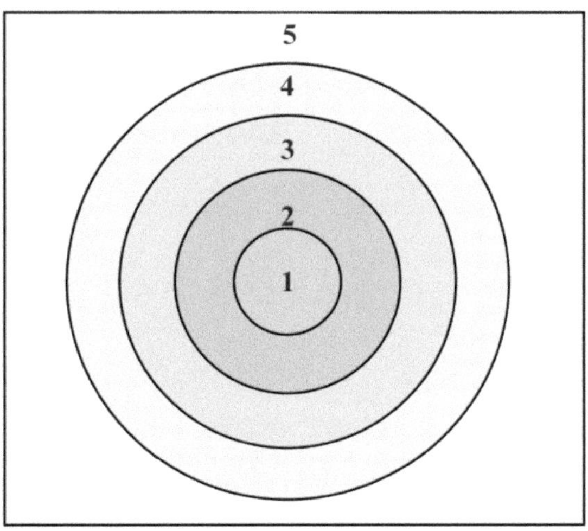

FIGURE 5.11 Body samples using different layers.

A bio-implantable spiral shape 3-D antenna was proposed for healthcare applications [26]. The antenna is compact with dimensions of 14×14×15 mm^3 as shown in Figure 5.12. To analyze the best spiral configuration, various shapes of the spiral were optimized at 405 MHz frequency. Further, by using the PIFA technique, the spiral antenna was miniaturized to the volume of 55% with only 1.4 dB loss in gain.

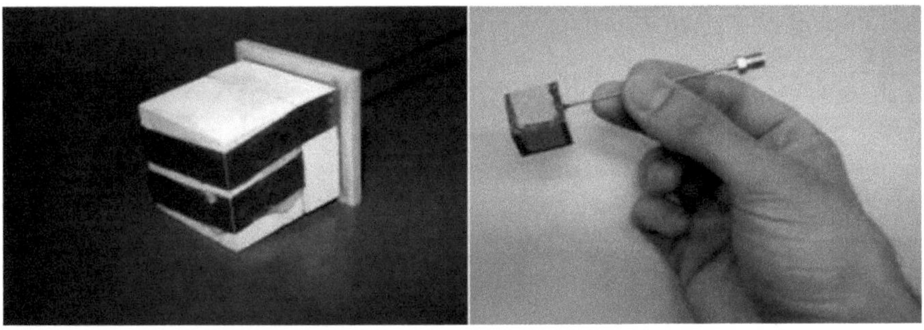

FIGURE 5.12 Photograph of the 3-D antenna [26].

In Ref. [27], a folded dipole antenna operating at 2.45 GHz ISM band was reported for biomedical applications as shown in Figure 5.13. The proposed antenna shows a wide bandwidth of around 50.2%. Two layers of antenna represented as superstate and substrate of material poly-dimethylsiloxane (PDMS) were used.

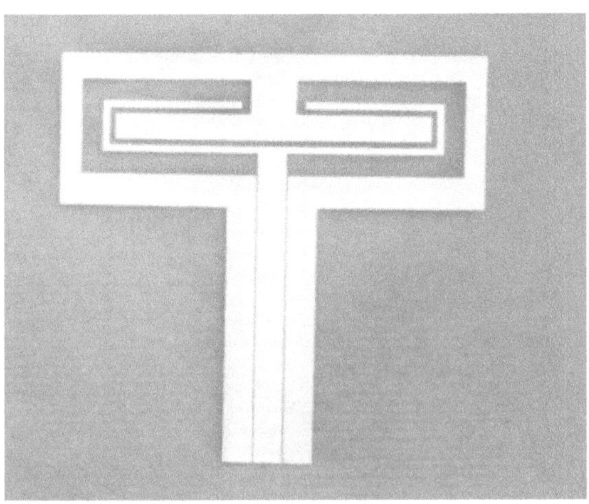

FIGURE 5.13 Photograph of the folded dipole antenna.

5.3 HEALTH CARE APPLICATIONS USING IOT

The area tends to the different medicinal services uses remote observing of patients, older care, remote drug, telemedicine, and giving consultancy through shrewd applications:

1. **Portable Individual Help:** This application makes the utilization of portable advances to empower remote access to current clinical frameworks or caregiving foundations. The brilliant versatile applications, entryways, sites, and so forth effectively accessible to all have made the mechanization of e-wellbeing frameworks simple [28].
2. **Keen Gadgets:** Smart gadgets in medicinal services are utilized to store and oversee key consideration parameters and to oversee the caught malady information. They are mainly sent for giving wellness arrangements by following objective exercises, demonstrative gadgets utilized for putting away information from gadgets. Essentially, they are utilized as wellness answers for following patient exercises and brilliant demonstrative gadgets. For example, pulse gadgets, pedometers, Google Glass, etc., utilized for catching the information from the sensors for further examination by a specialist.
3. **Telemedicine:** This application gives virtual help through a remote network and effective arrangements empowering virtual consideration interview, medication conveyance, and instruction. The determination of giving remote therapeutic help, for example, teleconferences, and versatile video arrangements have become extremely regular in a couple of nations and markets [29].
4. **Older Consideration:** This application clinically screens the maturing populace for making them autonomous. These gadgets incorporate wearable and embedded sensors for checking the older patients without requiring singular medication. The checking gadgets track the imperative indications of older consideration and transmit them to a standard cell phone which fills in as a hub for transmitting the continuous information to the specialists. The data consequently gathered can be utilized to give therapeutic help to the older folks and in the event of crises, close-by clinics can be alarmed [30].

5.4 HEALTHCARE SECURITY ISSUE IN IOT

So far as the examination work has been done, the security of the patient is of significant concern. The security prerequisites that appeared in Figure 5.14 should be satisfied so as to guarantee security in the IoT field. Likewise, because of the need-satisfying these security necessities, certain difficulties or issues that appeared in Figure 5.15 force enormous issues.

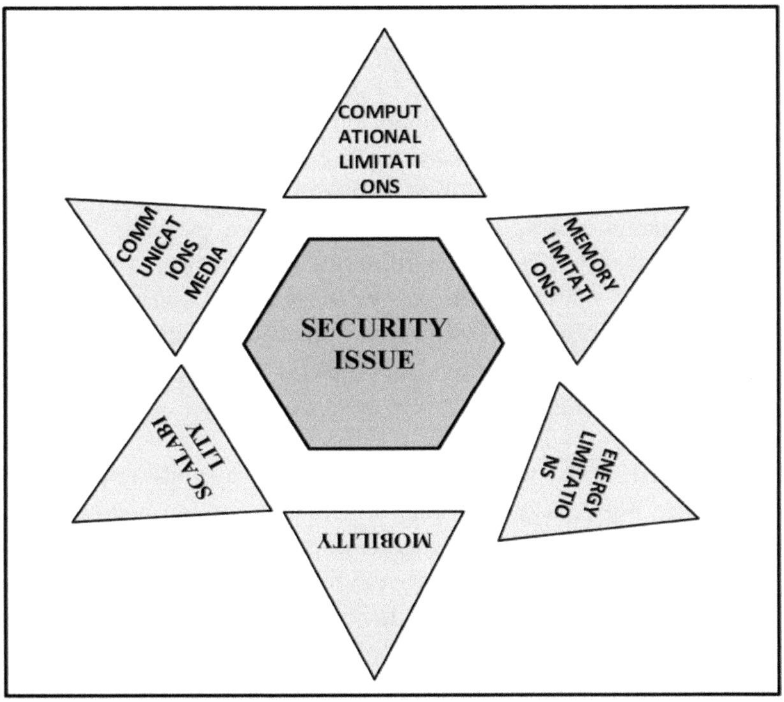

FIGURE 5.14 Security necessities in IoT healthcare.

Keen IoT gadgets are computationally compelled due to low-speed processors. These gadgets are intended for obliged situations performing cost in-effective tasks and for expanding their viability, security arrangement limiting asset utilization, and augmenting security is the need of an hour. The same is the case with memory calculation likewise as these gadgets do have a restricted on-gadget memory and consequently, as it were lightweight conventions or projects can be executed [31, 32].

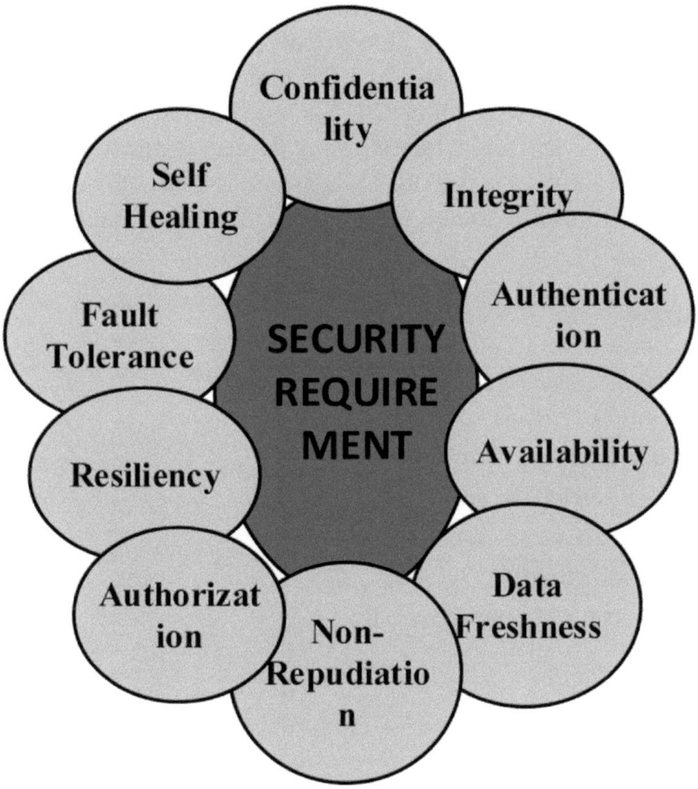

FIGURE 5.15 Security issues in IoT healthcare.

The savvy gadgets utilized in IoT social insurance, for example, blood weight sensor, temperature sensor have constrained battery power and along these lines spare power by initiating rest mode when no perusing should be accounted for. Subsequently, a viable structure arrangement ought to be actualized to bargain with the vitality, control, and computational impediment of these gadgets. Other security issues are identified with versatility [33, 34].

5.5 SUMMARY

This chapter discusses the need for wireless power transmission in today's life. Using this technology, researchers are collecting the RF energy, that is, freely available in the environment. After converting this RF energy, it shows great applications in the field of powering up of smart devices.

As explained in this chapter, the RF energy is used to power up the smart health care devices using IoT. This technique is also called green communication as the replacement of the device's battery is not required. This review features the possible ways and sources through which the researchers use the converted RF energy into the smart health care devices.

KEYWORDS

- **internet of things**
- **planar inverted-F antenna**
- **poly-dimethylsiloxane**
- **specific absorption rate**
- **ultra-wideband**
- **wireless body area networks**

REFERENCES

1. Laplante, P. A., & Laplante, N., (2016). The internet of things in healthcare: Potential applications and challenges. *IT Professional, 18*(3), 2–4.
2. Natarajan, K., Prasath, B., & Kokila, P., (2016). Smart healthcare system using internet of things. *Journal of Network Communications and Emerging Technologies, 6*(3), 37–42.
3. Singh, N., Kanaujia, B. K., Beg, M. T., Mainuddin, Khan, T., & Kumar, S., (2018). A dual polarized multiband rectenna for RF energy harvesting. *AEU-International Journal of Electronics and Communications, 93*, 123–131.
4. Singh, N., Kanaujia, B. K., Beg, M. T., Mainuddin, S. K., & Khandelwal, M. K., (2018). A dual band rectifying antenna for RF energy harvesting. *Journal of Computational Electronics, 17*(4), 1748–1755.
5. Al-Zuhairi, D. T., Gahl, J. M., Abed, A. M., & Islam, N. E., (2018). Characterizing Horn antenna signals for breast cancer detection. *Canadian Journal of Electrical and Computer Engineering, 41*(1), 8–16.
6. Lesnik, R., Verhovski, N., Mizrachi, I., Milgrom, B., & Haridim, M., (2018). Gain enhancement of a compact implantable dipole for biomedical applications. *IEEE Antennas and Wireless Propagation Letters, 17*(10), 1778–1782.

7. Abbasi, M. A. B., Nikolaou, S. S., Antoniades, M. A., NikolićStevanović, M., & Vryonides, P., (2017). Compact EBG-backed planar monopole for BAN wearable applications. *IEEE Transactions on Antennas and Propagation, 65*(2), 453–463.
8. Ashok, K. S., & Shanmuganantham, T., (2017). Design of clover slot antenna for biomedical applications. *Alexandria Engineering Journal, 56*(3), 313–317.
9. Liu, C., Guo, Y., & Xiao, S., (2014). Capacitively loaded circularly polarized implantable patch antenna for ISM band biomedical applications. *IEEE Transactions on Antennas and Propagation, 62*(5), 2407–2417.
10. Gandji, N. P., Lee, G., Semouchkin, G., Semouchkina, E., Neuberger, T., & Lanagan, M., (2019). Development and experimental testing of microstrip patch antenna-inspired RF probes for 14-T MRI scanners. *IEEE Transactions on Microwave Theory and Techniques, 67*(1), 443–453.
11. Shah, I. A., Zada, M., & Yoo, H., (2019). Design and analysis of a compact-sized multiband spiral-shaped implantable antenna for scalp implantable and leadless pace-maker systems. *IEEE Transactions on Antennas and Propagation, 67*(6), 4230–4234.
12. Xu, L., Bo, Y., Lu, W., Zhu, L., & Guo, C., (2019). Circularly polarized annular ring antenna with wide axial-ratio bandwidth for biomedical applications. *IEEE Access, 7*, 59999–60009.
13. Singh, N., Kanaujia, B. K., Beg, M. T., Mainuddin, S. K., Choi, H. C., & Kim, K. W., (2019). Low profile multiband rectenna for efficient energy harvesting at microwave frequencies. *International Journal of Electronics*. doi:10.1080/ 00207217.2019.1636302.
14. Brown, W. C., (1984). The history of power transmission by radio waves. *IEEE Transactions on Microwave Theory and Techniques, 32*(9), 1230–1242.
15. Salonen, P., Rahmat-Samii, Y., Hurme, H., & Kivikoski, M., (2004). Dual band wearable textile antenna. *IEEE Antennas and Propagation Society Symposium* (Vol. 1, pp. 463–466). Monterey, CA, USA.
16. Soontornpipit, P., Furse, C., & Chung, Y. C., (2004). Design of implantable micro strip antenna for communication with medical implants. *IEEE Transactions on Microwave Theory and Techniques, 52*, 1944–1951.
17. Dobbins, J. A., Chu, A. W., Fink, P. W., Kennedy, T. F., Lin, G. Y., Khayat, M. A., & Scully, R. C., (2006). Fabric equiangular spiral antenna. *IEEE Antennas and Propagation Society International Symposium* (pp. 2113–2116). Albuquerque, NM.
18. Soh, P. J., Vandenbosch, G. A. E., Ooi, S. L., & Rais, N. H. M., (2012). Design of broadband all-textile slotted PIFA. *IEEE Transactions on Antennas and Propagation, 60*(1), 379–384.
19. Salonen, P., & Rantanen, J., (2001). A dual band and wide-band antenna on flexible substrate for smart clothing. In: *27th Annual Conference of the IEEE* (Vol. 1).
20. Nikolova, K. N., (2003). *Antenna Lectures*. McMaster University, Hamilton, ON, Canada.
21. Osman, M. A. R., Abd, R. M. K., Samsuri, N. A., Salim, H. A. M., & Ali, M. F., (2011). Embroidered fully textile wearable antenna for medical monitoring applications. *Progress in Electromagnetics Research, 117*, 321–337.
22. Klemm, M., Locher, I., & Troster, G., (2004). A novel circularly polarized textile antenna for wearable applications. In: *34th European Microwave Conference* (pp. 137–140). Amsterdam, the Netherlands.

23. Khaleel, H. R., Al-Rizzo, H. M., Rucker, D. G., & Elwi, T. A., (2010). Wearable yagi micro strip antenna for telemedicine applications. *Proceedings of the 2010 IEEE Radio and Wireless Symposium* (pp. 280–283). New Orleans, LA.
24. Hertleer, C., Rogier, H., & Van, L. L., (2007). A textile antenna for protective clothing. *IET Seminar on Antennas and Propagation for Body-Centric Wireless Communications* (pp. 44–46). London.
25. Merli, F., Fuchs, B., Mosig, J. R., & Skrivervik, A. K., (2011). The effect of insulating layers on the performance of implanted antennas. *IEEE Transactions on Antennas and Propagation, 59*(1), 21–31.
26. Abadia, J., Merli, F., Zurcher, J. F., Mosig, J. R., & Skrivervik, A. K., (2009). 3D-spiral small antenna design and realization for biomedical telemetry in the MICS band. *Radio Engineering, 18*(4), 359–367.
27. Lucia, M., Kurup, D., Rogier, H., Ginste, D. V., Axisa, F., Vanfleteren, J., Joseph, W., Martens, L., & Vermeeren, G., (2011). Design of an implantable slot dipole conformal flexible antenna for biomedical applications. *IEEE Transactions on Antennas and Propagation, 59*(10), 3556–3564.
28. Riazul, I. S. M., Humaun, K. M. D., Kwak, D., Kyung-Sup, K., & Mahmud, H., (2015). *The Internet of Things for Health Care: A Comprehensive Survey*. doi: 10.1109/ACCESS.2015.2437951.
29. Ovidiu Vermesan & Peter Friess, (2014). *Internet of Things: From Research and Innovation to Market Deployment-IERC*. https://www.researchgate.net/publication/263970385_Internet_of_Things_From_Research_and_Innovation_to_Market_Deployment_Chapter_4_-_Internet_of_Things_Global_Standardisation_-_State_of_Play (accessed on 29 July 2020).
30. Li, C., Raghunathan, A., & Jha, N., (2011). Hijacking an insulin pump: Security attacks and defenses for a diabetes therapy system. In: *IEEE 13th International Conference on eHealth Networking, Applications, and Services* (pp. 150–156). Columbia, MO.
31. Christin, D., Reinhardt, A., Mogre, P., & Steinmed, R., (2009). Wireless sensor networks and the internet of things: Selected challenges. In: *Proceedings of the 8th GI/ITG KuVS Fachgespräch "Drahtlose Sensornede"* (pp. 31–33).
32. Xu, X., Zhou, J., & Wang, H., (2013). Research on the basic characteristics, the key technologies, and the network architecture and security problems of the internet of things. In: *3rd International Conference on Computer Science and Network Technology*.
33. Riazulislam, S. M., Daehan, K., Humaun, K. M., Mahmud, H., & Kyung-Sup, K., (2015). The internet of things for health care: A comprehensive survey. *IEEE Access*.
34. Pang, Z., Tian, J., & Chen, Q., (2014). Intelligent packaging and intelligent medicine box for medication management towards the internet-of-things. In: *Proc. 16th International Conference in Advance Communication Technology (ICACT)*.
35. Linklabs (2015). *IoT in Health Care: What You Should Know,* December 23, 2015. (Online) Available: https://www.link-labs.com/blog/IoT-in-healthcare (accessed on 13 August 2020).

CHAPTER 6

Image and Signal Processing in E-Health Applications

DIVYA PRAKASH PATTANAYAK and SURYA PRAKASH PATTANAYAK

Department of Electronics and Communication, Ambedkar Institute of Advanced Communication Technologies and Research, New Delhi, India, E-mail: suryankbabu@gmail.com (S. P. Pattanayak)

ABSTRACT

Signal processing is associated with the representation of signals by a sequence of numbers or symbols and the processing of these signals. Digital signal processing is a branch of science which deals with signal processing. It includes areas like audio, speech, sonar, and radar signal processing, sensor array processing, spectral estimation, signal processing for communications, statistical signal processing, digital image processing, control of systems, biomedical signal processing, seismic data processing, etc.

Biomedical signals are the recording of observations due to physiological activities of organisms, ranging from gene and protein sequences to neural and cardiac rhythms–to tissue and organ images. It is a clinical study of the internal body metabolisms, diagnosis of ailments, and detection of diseases using the electronic instrumentation. Signal processing aims at extracting significant information from biomedical signals. With the aid of biomedical signal processing, biologists can discover new biology and physicians can monitor the distinct illness.

Signal processing came into the field of medical signal processing (MSP) with the advent use of advanced electronic instruments in the biomedical field. Various scientists invented many instruments that detected the biological diagnostic resulted from biological organisms. MSP has enabled the people from the medical field to enable them to ease off their burdens of life support in a very healthy manner. While these techniques are well established, the field of MSP continues to expand thanks to the invention and development of various novel biomedical instruments.

6.1 INTRODUCTION

Digital imaging is the process of constructing an image from applied signals of different types. Object classification of these images can be done in multiple ways, that is, radiation pattern, the field used, characteristics to be investigated, and direct or indirect. Medical imaging is a procedural technique to study various properties of the human body, organ, and tissue by accessing various signals from the body. It includes medical imaging and processing. Output results can be of two types analog and discrete. Discrete images can be further simplified by digital images by the process of digitization. The main difficulties and challenges associated with it are an accurate interpretation of input signal, efficient analysis, and derivative of optimum diagnostic information of the image.

6.1.1 DIGITAL IMAGE PROCESSING SYSTEM

A complete digital process imaging system is a collection of hardware and software equipment. It acquires image information by use of available appropriate sensor and captures the characteristics of interest from the object in the best suitable way. If the required image is analog in nature, it is digitized by analog to digital converter (ADC), after images stored in permanent or temporary in memory which includes RAM, ROM, floppy disk, flash memory, and CD's. In the processing stage of digital image processing, image manipulation and derivation of desired results are obtained by proper utilization of image processing techniques so as to reach an efficient diagnostic procedure.

The final outcome image displayed on the computer monitor TV or film this action requires the conversion of analog data to digital data using an ADC. Image enhancement results in the image which is produced from the base image after the application of several enhancement techniques; to adjust its brightness, contrast, and shade. Smoothing of noise, speckle, and as well as sharpening of the image are also done. The enhancement procedure aims to make the image more informative easily understandable and improvise to derive the information from it. The image restoration procedure is used to reverse the degradation of the image. It includes the reversing effect of uneven illumination, non-linear detection, distortion, poor focus, unwanted noise, speckle, etc. (Figure 6.1).

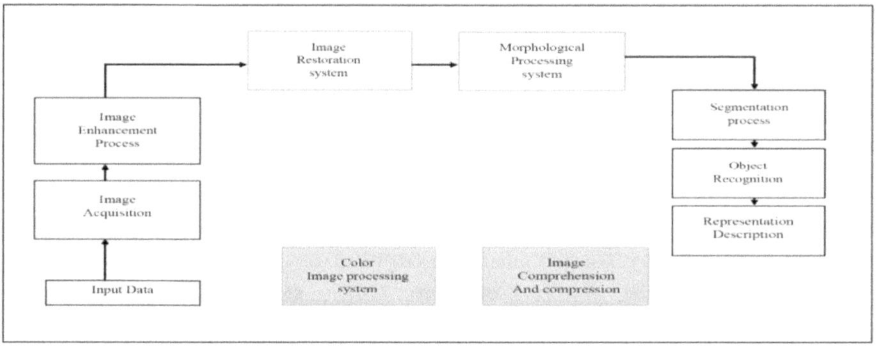

FIGURE 6.1 Digital image processing system.

6.1.2 *IMAGE ANALYSIS*

The image analysis process involves grouping and classification. Normally it starts isolation from the area of interest to the rest of the image (image segmentation). Image feature includes size, shape, and texture which are classified into groups according to their characteristics.

These classifications of an object depend on the tolerance level of a grouping which is done either fall into a group or includes into the group (the tolerance level is set by the user or radiologist). In further classification process, pattern recognition is done to recognize the cluster benign and malignant area in the image. It is the best technique for cancer detection or oncology.

6.1.3 *IMAGE COMPRESSION*

Image compression reduces the size of the image and data required to describe the particular image. Compression of the image leads to the saving of data in storage memory and more information to be stored in the same available data memory. The compression of the image is done without any loss of information as their area may be repetitive and redundant in a given image. Removal of this redundant and repetitive area does not hamper the desired information of the image and overall compression is done without information loss.

Some of the important compression techniques of digital image processing are loss and lossless compression.

6.1.4 IMAGE SYNTHESIS

Image synthesis is a process of creating a new image from the available image or non-image information. For example, reconstruction of axial or slices tomography from x and y computed projection. The data image processing technique consists of correctly followed step-by-step procedures to extract the data from the area of interest. Often it is performed sequentially but in case of more complicated data, extraction feedback mechanisms are also utilized. Sometimes even iterative loop is used to refine the extracted information.

6.1.5 APPLICATIONS

It includes MRI, ultrasound, laparoscopy, angiography, Doppler imaging, mammography, Doppler imaging, EEG, and ECG.

6.2 MRI

Magnetic resonance imaging (MRI) is a non-ionizing technique that uses radiofrequency (200 MHz–2 GHz) electromagnetic (EM) radiation and large magnetic fields (around 1–2 tesla (T), compared with the Earth's magnetic field of about 0.5×10^{-4} T) [1]. This large magnetic field radiation is created by a very good quality of superconductivity magnets into which current is passed through superconducting lines having resistance almost zero. Images created in MRI provide detail physiological and anatomical structure of the body with a three-dimensional feature with perfect visualization of soft tissue.

6.2.1 NUCLEAR MRI

MRI images can be obtained from the NMR spectrum. In the case of a particular tissue, it remains in two different positions. NMR spectrum beam would produce a single distortion for it. Investigation of the produced spectrum would show the presence of protons but will not provide their definite location. In addition to the magnetic field, superconductivity electromagnet produces a linear magnetic field gradient using an electromagnet coil to develop a small gradient of Milli tesla which is also applied leading to an increased magnetic field across the study area. As the Larmor frequency directly proportional to the applied magnetic field, it is quite different for the same tissue located at different positions of the body leading FID signal to be complicated.

For the two voxels at different positions, the Fourier transform of the FID signal will produce two distortions for two voxels, one for each voxel. These two distortions have spatial information and produce a spectrum. Spectrum is considered as projection very much similar to X-ray computed tomography (CT). Multiple projections around the study area of patient tissue lead to the reconstruction of the axial image. The slice selection is done by using frequency selected radiofrequency pulses.

When radiologists apply simultaneously one of the magnetic field gradients, the choice of X, Y, Z gradient are selected to obtain the required orientation of the image. The slice thickness position is varied by using different radio frequency bandwidth. But there is a limit to it, as to how can it be sliced smaller value of bandwidth and large value of the magnetic field is difficult to generate. Also, thin slices contain few spins and a very small SNR. By changing the central frequency of the radiofrequency pulse, a particular slice can be moved to different position of the study area.

To produce two-dimensional image, X and Y direction and encoding of the slices, the direction encoding is done by frequency change during acquisition. The column of a pixel is formed left to right so as to discriminate in terms of different frequencies that occur known as frequency encoding.

Gradient application in the y-direction to change the frequency in the dimension is not enough to describe each color of a pixel. A number of gradients are necessary to produce phase change before acquisition Fourier transform provides enough data to encode the final images called phase encoding. Three separated gradient calls are necessary for three spatial dimensions multiple projections can be obtained by rotating the magnetic field over the study area.

Fourier transform of the signal echo received from the object in a certain direction effectively produce a projected image. One-dimensional projection, two-dimensional Fourier transform of the object, later inverse Fourier transform produces the axial image. The whole process is done by Direct Fourier transform reconstruction technique (DFR).

6.2.2 MRI SYSTEM

It is a universally accepted MRI reconstruction technique. The main component of the MRI scanner is shown in Figure 6.2; primary magnet polarizer protons.

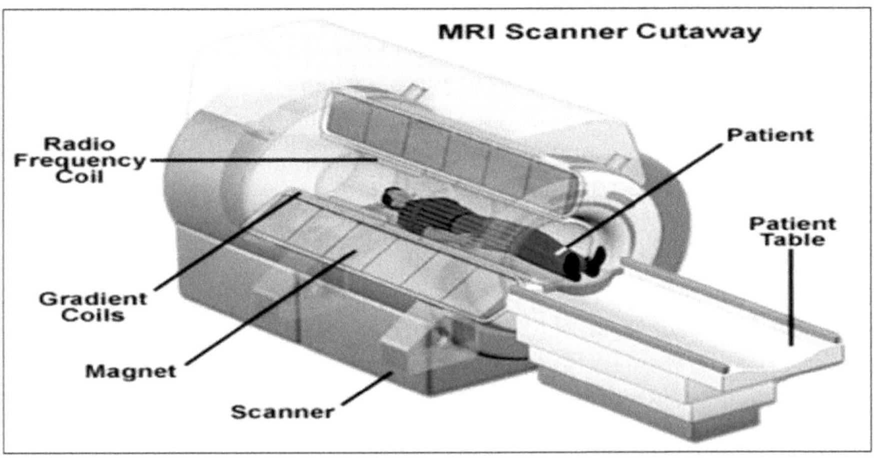

FIGURE 6.2 Magnetic resonance imaging scanner system.

The gradient coil produces magnetic field linear variation in which proton starts recreation at a particular frequency within the patient's body. The radiofrequency coil develops an oscillating magnetic field to produce phase coherence and receive. FID signals by the process of magnetic induction are kept around the study area of the patient's body to be imaged (Figure 6.3).

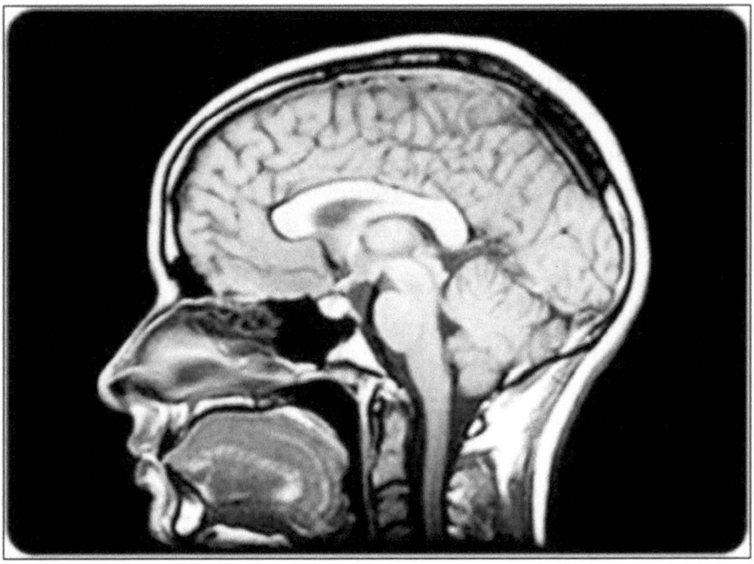

FIGURE 6.3 The slice image of the brain in magnetic resonance imaging.

6.2.3 ADVANTAGES

MRI does not use the radiation and hence non-invasive in nature produce safe intensity has a low risk to the person. MRI does not produce an allergic reaction, which occurs by iodine. Chemical substances are not used in techniques of x-rays and CT scans.

6.2.4 DISADVANTAGES

In the MRI technique, it uses a magnetic field so the metallic items are not appropriate during a medical procedure. People who have pacemakers and other medical gadgets like knee caps are not able to carry the test.

6.2.5 APPLICATION

MRI is widely used in studying the affected area of the brain as well as used in scanning the abdominal pelvic region. MRI is also used in imaging of cardiovascular, neuroimaging, musculoskeletal, and liver gastrointestinal (GI) tract.

6.3 ANGIOGRAPHY

Angiography is a technique used to examine tissues, blood vessels, and lumen of the affected area. In this process wire cables containing contrast attributes at its end which is inserted into the patient's body. It absorbs the x-ray and shows the picture inside the blood vessel. It is widely used in the diagnosis of coronary heart diseases. As in the world, millions of people die due to heart disease. Narrowing of blood vessels which affects the oxygen-carrying capacity of the blood to. There are various types of angiography such as cerebral, peripheral, neurovascular, coronary, and fluorescein.

6.3.1 WORKING

Coronary artery disease is a leading heart disease-causing numerous deaths worldwide. It happens when a coronary artery supplying the blood becomes hard, stiff, and narrow. It generally occurs as fats get deposited in the inner walls of the vessel. According to time, this fat deposition increases in size. As a result, Lumen starts decreasing leading to less blood flow and the heart receives less oxygenated blood. Hence results in a mycobacterial infraction and heart attack which causes permanent damage to heart muscles. The main goals of angiography are to visualize coronary arteries, branches, collaterals, and anomalies, precise localization relative to major and minor side branches, thrombi, and areas of calcification and to visualize vessel bifurcations, the origin of side branches, and specific lesion characteristics (length, eccentricity, calcium, etc.).

In this wire, the cable is inserted into the patients' body which absorbs the x-ray to make blood vessels visible. The images are then obtained on TV or monitor called digital image subtraction technique. In this, it nullifies the images of bones and other tissues only shows the desired blood vessels (Figure 6.4).

6.3.2 FLUORESCENT ANGIOGRAPHY

In this technique, the special fluorescent dye is inserted into blood vessels and it radiates and shows the particular vessels used in the diagnosis of affected areas. Generally, this technique is used in the diagnosis of damaged blood vessels of eyes (Figure 6.5).

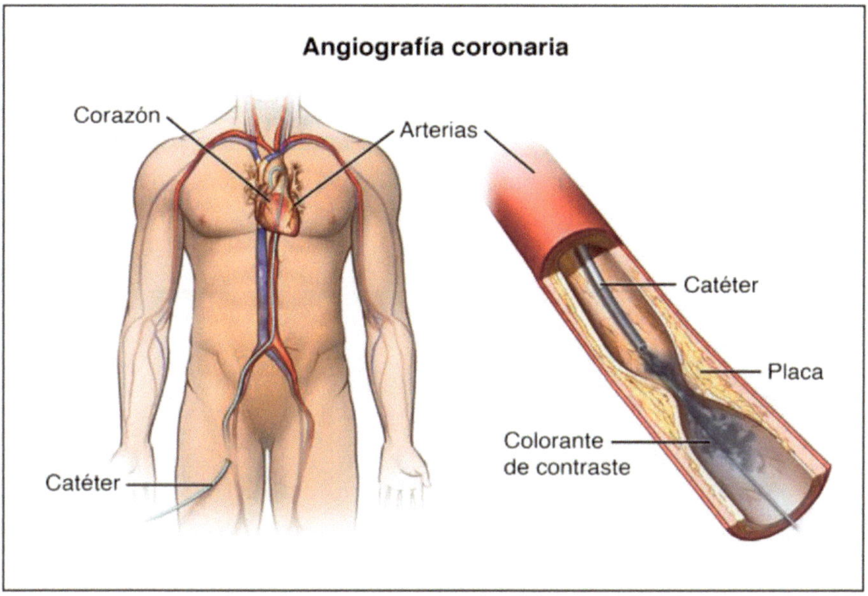

FIGURE 6.4 A coronary angiography procedure.

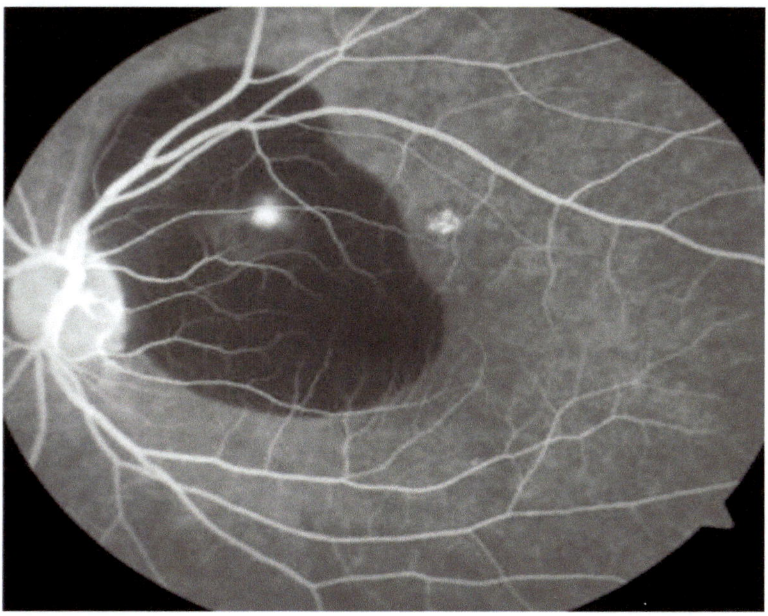

FIGURE 6.5 Fluorescent angiography showing eye blood vessels.

6.3.3 NEUROVASCULAR ANGIOGRAPHY

In this technique generally, the blood vessels carrying oxygenated blood and deoxygenated blood to the brain are analyzed and examined. It is based on the principle of the image subtraction method. In which it nullifies the bones and other tissues and frames of an image are taken and combined to form a single image on the monitor (Figure 6.6).

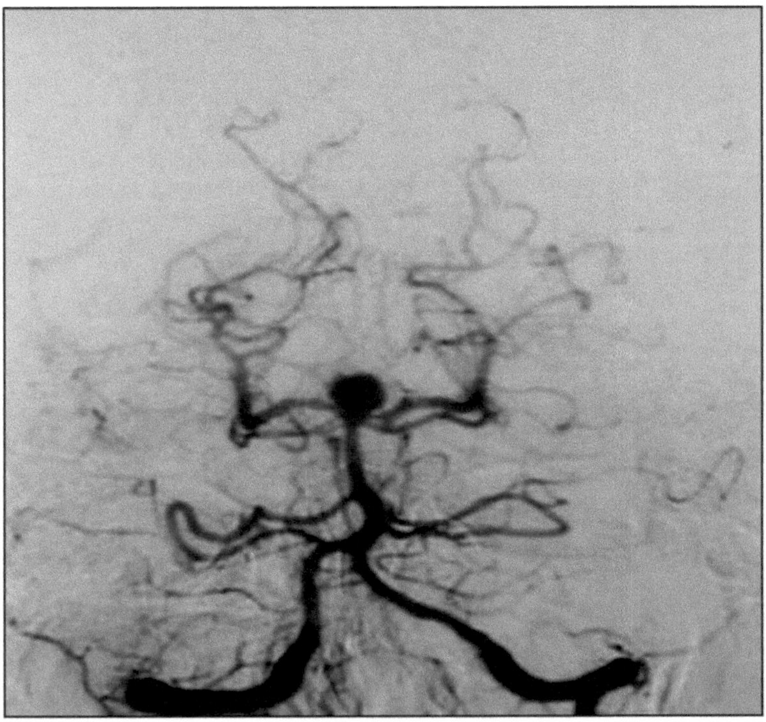

FIGURE 6.6 Neurovascular angiography.

6.3.4 PERIPHERAL ANGIOGRAPHY

In this, the patient suffering from renal stenosis which results in stroke due to the narrowing of blood vessels. In this technique, the narrowing vessel in the legs is examined and treated by angiography through the artery (Figure 6.7).

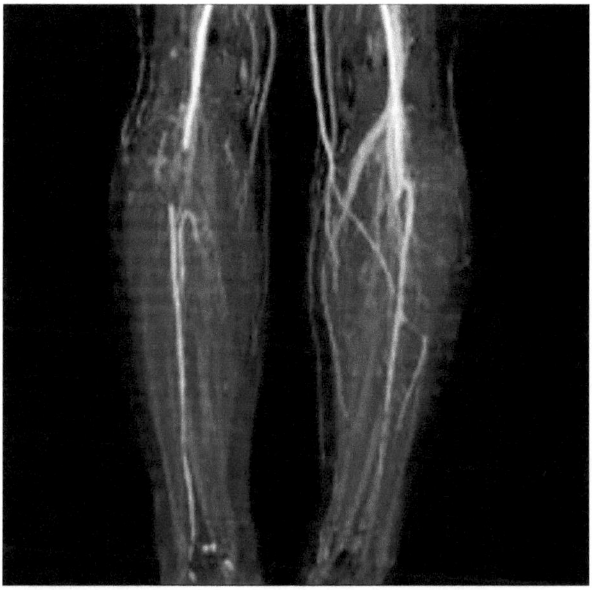

FIGURE 6.7 The blood capillaries of peripheral angiography in legs.

6.3.5 CEREBRAL ANGIOGRAPHY

Many complicated cases are due to strokes, seizures, and hemorrhage which occurs due to damaging of vessels in the brain. An angiogram can also be used to help treat some of the conditions involving the blood vessels of the neck and brain [2]. Brain vessels are analyzed and examined for the affected area of interest. It also uses the digital image subtraction technique (Figure 6.8).

6.3.6 ADVANTAGES

It is more precise, small blood vessels are located easily and accurately than other imaging techniques.

6.3.7 DISADVANTAGES

In this process, there is a chance of complication. The complication is such as renal failure, embolization, and thrombosis. This procedure requires the blood bleeding to carry the test. This procedure is case sensitive in case of a person suffering from diabetes and thalassemia in which bleeding does not stop easily.

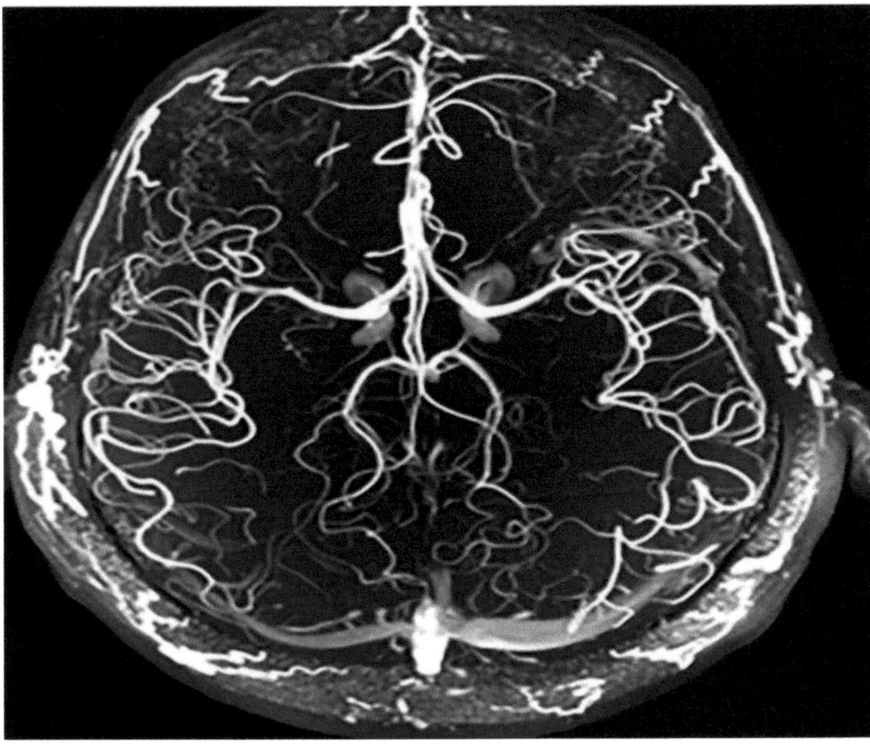

FIGURE 6.8 Cerebral angiography in the human brain.

Source: Adapted from: Figure 3 [2].

6.4 ULTRASOUND

Ultrasonic imaging uses high-frequency (~1–10 MHz) sound waves and their echoes to produce images that can demonstrate organ movement in real-time [1]. The high-frequency wave is transmitted to the desired area and a cross-section image is formed from the received intensity of echoes. Ultrasound imaging technique uses an envelope detection principle so it only provides the intensity of information. In spite of the drawbacks, it is widely used in medical imaging as it produces a real-time image of the human body at a low cost. Ultrasound waves are not invasive and non-ionizing modality; therefore, it has a low risk to the person undergoing diagnostic (Figure 6.9).

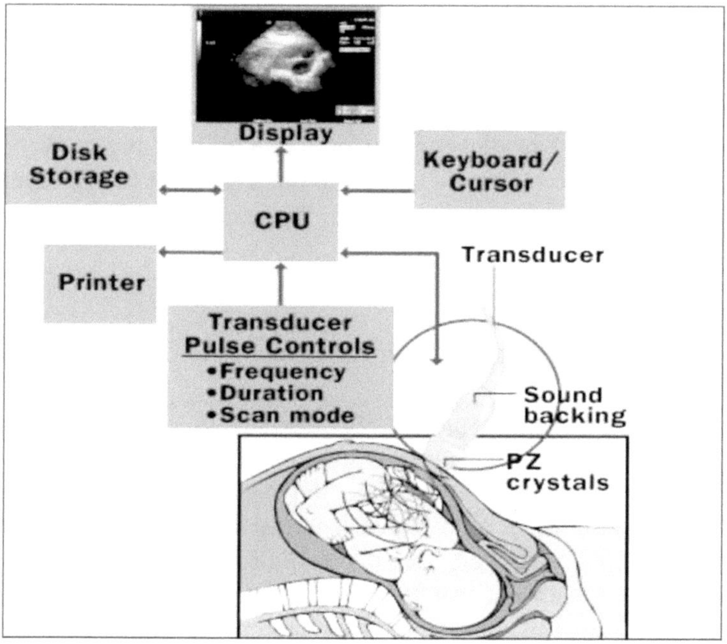

FIGURE 6.9 Ultrasound imaging system.

6.4.1 *WORKING*

In the medical ultrasound imaging, high-frequency sound waves (1 to 10 megahertz) are transmitted and the echoes are received to form a real-time image of human tissue. The transducer probe generates and receives sound waves using a principle called the piezoelectric (pressure electricity) effect, which was discovered by Pierre and Jacques Curie in 1880 [9]. Ultrasound transducer consists of a piezoelectric crystal of lead zirconate titanate (PZT) which is embedded between the two electrodes to produce 1 to 5 microsecond long pulses The Crystal starts resonating when a small sinusoidal voltage applied to it. The sound waves produced on its surface travels forward and backward). Generally, pulses are separated by 1 ms, which results in a pulse repetition rate of 1000 Hz due to which they flow through the soft tissue at a speed of 1540 m s^{-1} with respect to the speed of sound 330 m s^{-1} as a longitudinal wave. In the body different tissues, have different acoustical properties due to which fraction of the waves are reflected and detected by the crystal. The ultrasound image forms only that part of the image where the waves are reflected about 180 degrees from the transmitted signal. The depth of the attribute can be measured by determining a delay between the pulse reception and transmission. The speed of propagation and brightness image is determined by the intensity of the Echo detected by the transducer. The depth of the picture can be determined by echoes of sound waves on the basis of A (amplitude)-mode of ultrasound. This is generally used for the diagnosis of liver cirrhosis, myocardial infarction, and eye tumor.

6.4.2 IMAGE QUALITY OF ULTRASOUND

The image quality depends on the reflected distinct signals between the close separations of two attributes which must be equal to half the spatial pulse length. The axial resolution is better when shorter pulses are used. Generally, a spatial resolution which is parallel to propagation ultrawave is known as axial resolution. Lateral resolution is 90 degrees to that of the direction of ultrasound waves. It is measured from the diffraction of an ultrasonic beam from its initial cross-section size. The Beam diverges to $\sin^{-1}$ (1.2 λ/w), where w is the diameter of the transducer due to the diffraction. It also lowers down the energy of the main beam as the side lobe increases and introduces the artifacts of the image. SNR of the reflected signal depends on the bandwidth and intensity of the ultrasound pulse. So the ultrasound transducer is focused primarily on the tissue to have a better image. SNR drops to 2.0 if the speckle from small inhomogeneities is included. The contrast of image is enhanced using a small gas field microsphere for microbubble having a diameter less than 10 micrometers into the blood vessels which increase the reflected echo from the tissues.

Also, the image quality is affected by bone as it has high attenuation coefficient. The transmission of an ultrasonic wave in the bone is minimum so reverberations occur inside the patient's body. Bones and air act as a strong reflector which causes bright-line spots in an image. Image shadowing also occurs when there is a high reflector for a higher attenuating substance is present.

6.4.3 *THE TWO-DIMENSIONAL TOMOGRAPHY*

The two-dimensional tomography or B brightness mode is a more common way to produce the anatomical image. In this method, the ultrasound transducer is repeatedly moved all over the patient's body to get the maximum reflected signals by correcting the attenuation path. The beam is swept back and forth from brighter dots. The sweeping beam produces a series of brighter dots from a single vertical line by each sweep. The beam steering can be done manually or electronically array of piezoelectric crystal elements. When all the echoes are produced along a particular beam direction, the time delay is introduced into the array elements due to which the second line data is acquired (Figure 6.10).

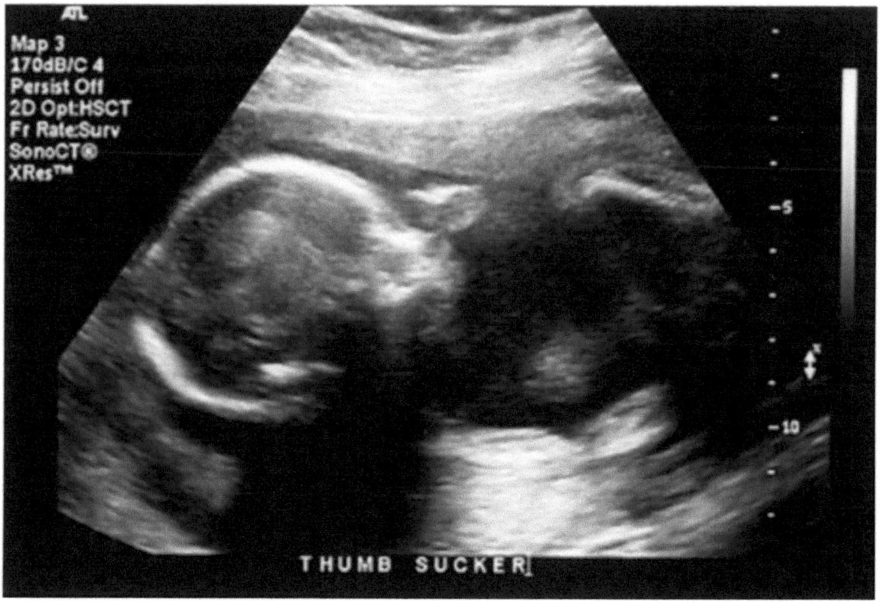

FIGURE 6.10 The B mode image scans of the fetus.

6.4.4 *THREE-DIMENSIONAL ULTRASOUND*

Imaging is obtained by using additional rows piezoelectric crystal elements, which have direction perpendicular to the B mode scan. If a smaller number of rows are added only a limited area swept and a large number of rows are added the array is two dimensional and the sweeping beam makes three-dimensional images. It includes detection of the tumor, study fetus, and uterine malformation (Figure 6.11).

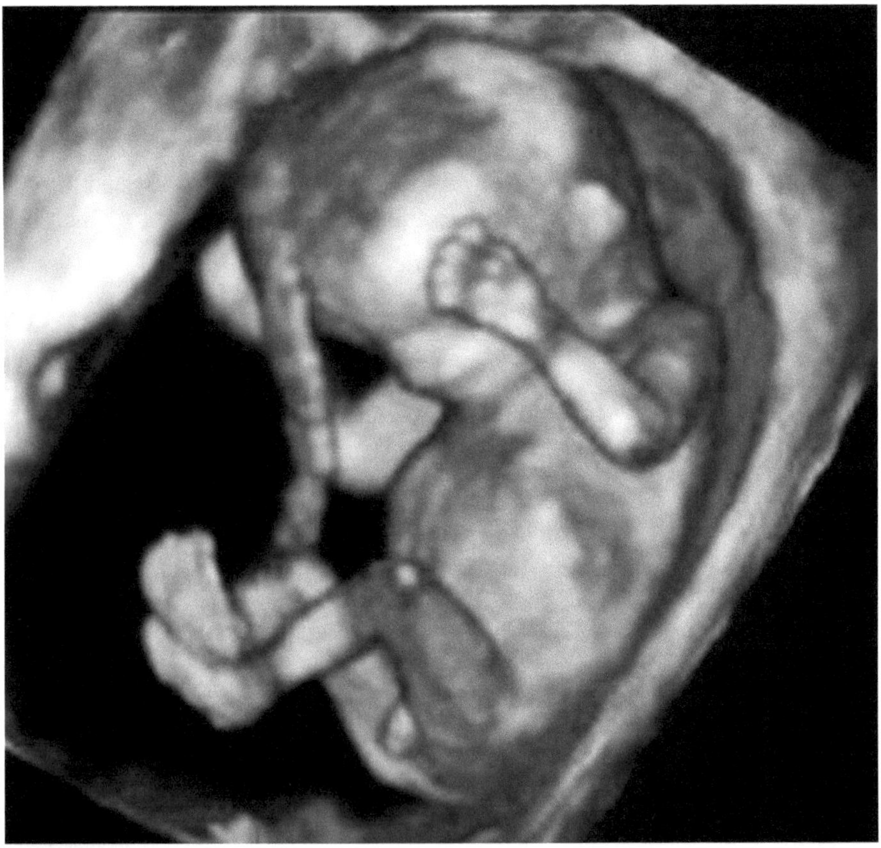

FIGURE 6.11 The three-dimensional image scan of 12 weeks fetus.

6.4.5 *ADVANTAGES*

The patients are exposed to the non-ionizing radiation and thus it has low risk to the patients. In this technique, it also does not require the incision, cut, needles, bleeding, or anesthesia. Hence, it is painless and comfortable to carry out procedures. It is less expensive and accurate in locating soft tissues.

6.4.6 DISADVANTAGES

It requires a skilled and expert operator. The bowel of the patient should be filled with water, not air as air prevents reflections. It takes a longer time in imaging. It has poor penetration in bone and hence shadowing effect occurs.

6.5 WHAT IS DOPPLER IMAGING?

Medical Doppler imaging technique is based on the principle of the Doppler effect. It is a variation in frequency or pitch of a wave in relation to the observer moving relative to the sound source. It is used to measure the blood velocity in the arteries mainly the diagnosis of stenosis, cardiac output, and narrowing of arteries (Figure 6.12).

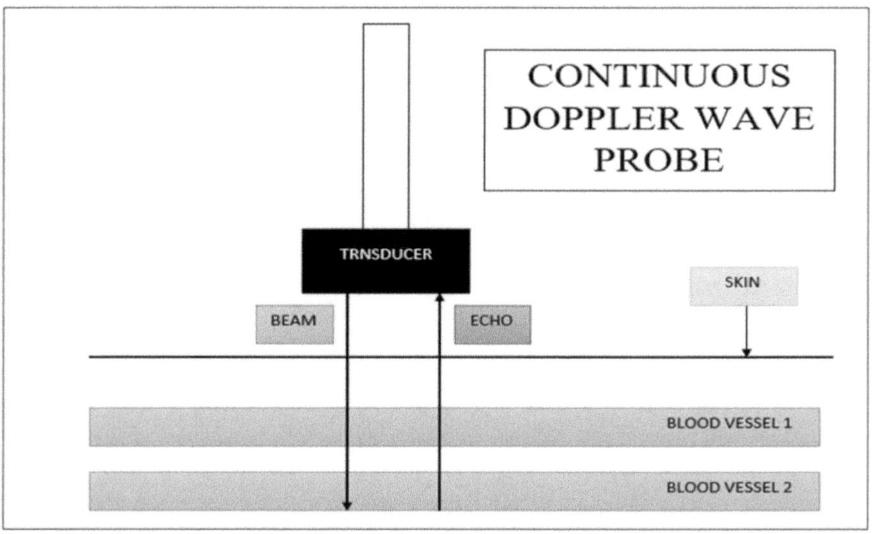

FIGURE 6.12 Doppler imaging system.

6.5.1 WORKING

Doppler imaging technique consists of two crystals in the transducer used for transmitting and receiving sound waves. When the RBC moving towards the transducer receives high frequency due to velocity, both transducer and RBC act as a sound source. The signals are scattered in every direction and reflected are Doppler shifted twice. These differences can be measured as a direct time difference or, more usually, in terms of a phase shift from which the 'Doppler frequency' [8].

The reflected signal is amplified and mixed with a transmitted signal and the difference signal applied to the spectrum analyzer to determine the Doppler Shift. The angle is determined by the B mode scan. Color flow imaging can be used to identify vessels requiring examination, to identify the presence and direction of flow, to highlight gross circulation anomalies, throughout the entire color flow image, and to provide beam/ vessel angle correction for velocity measurements [3]. The most common Doppler medical imaging mapping technique is BART. When the RBC is moving away from the transducer, it is considered as blue and moving towards the transducer it is considered as red (Figure 6.13).

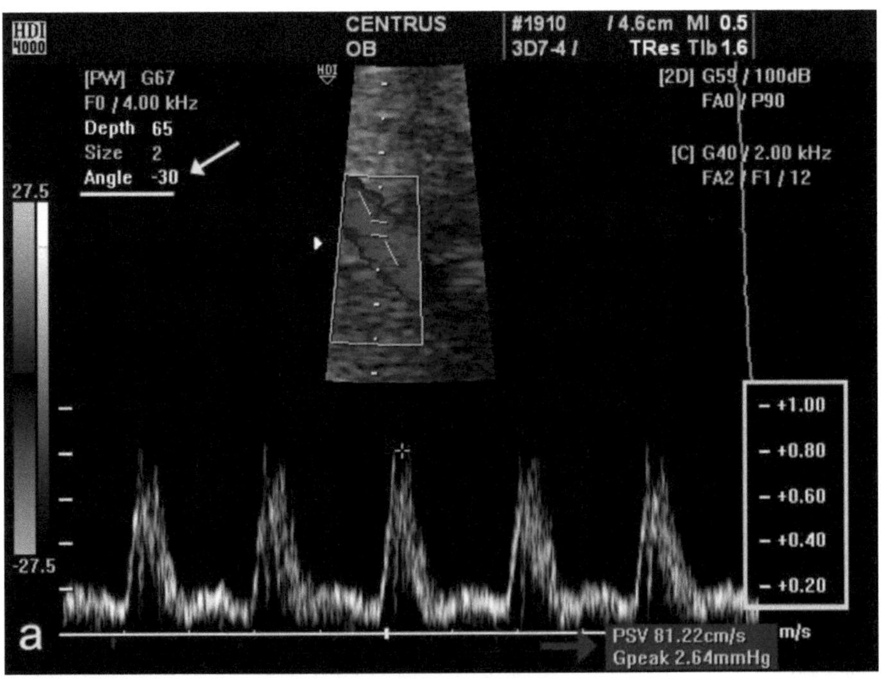

FIGURE 6.13 Two dimensional spectral Doppler plots.

6.5.2 ADVANTAGES

In Doppler imaging technique, patients are exhibited to the non-ionizing electromagnetic radiations, i.e., lower risk to the patients. In this methodology, there is no requirement of incisions, cuts, needles, and anesthesia. In consequence, it is bleeding less, painless, and comfortable medical procedure. It is less expensive and the velocity of blood can be measured.

6.5.3 DISADVANTAGES

The speed of particles, strong reflection, and scattering can make a false analysis. The speed is variable in the liquid part and it requires an expert and skilled radiologists for maneuvering.

6.6 MAMMOGRAPHY

Mammography is the technique of detecting breast cancer among women using low-intensity x-ray. The main objective is to detect cancer at an early stage so that chemotherapy or surgery can be operative. In this process, human tissue is exposed to low energy radiation of(17.5 to 19.6 eV) to form images inside the body. The images are then examined for microcalcification or any type of lumps. The most common and oldest form of imaging are X-rays. Today, advanced technologies includes digital mammography, CAD, and 3D mammography (tomosynthesis) (Figure 6.14).

6.6.1 DIGITAL MAMMOGRAPH

Digital mammography uses digital receptors which are substituted in place of conventional x-ray film the electrical signals. The signals are then analyzed on the computer screen which provides better resolution and image manipulation. The computer-aided detection (CAD) involves segmentation in image processing. As CAD increases the efficiency of detection by allocating free adding mammograms to abnormal areas and alerting the lab technician to examine the area. The digitized images may indicate the presence of cancer by examining the microcalcification mass and density of the tissue.

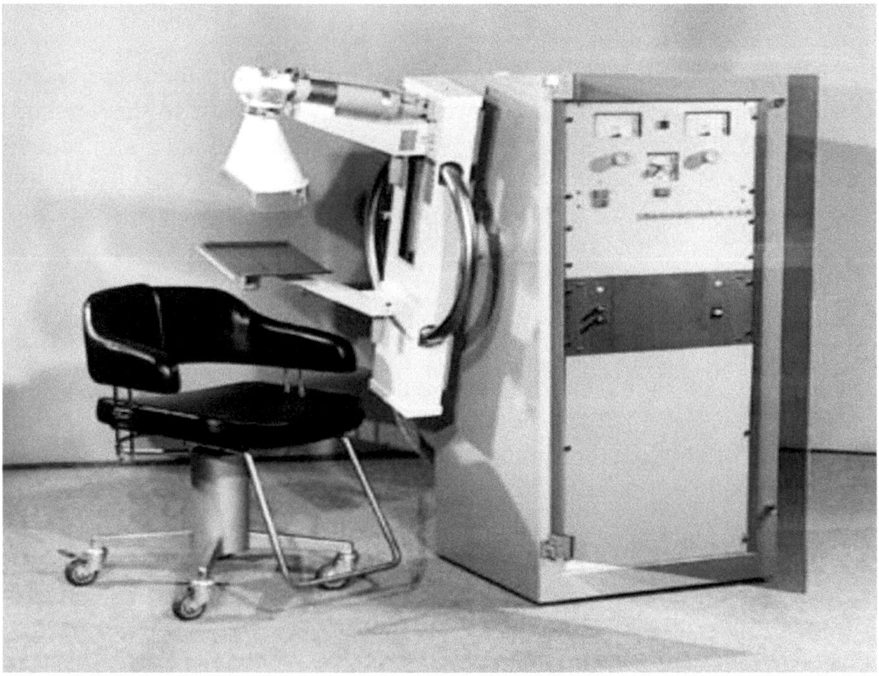

FIGURE 6.14 Mammography system.

6.6.2 3D MAMMOGRAPHY

3D mammography of breast tomosynthesis in this technique the multiple images from various angles are produced and synthesized to form a three-dimensional image. 3D tomography involves breast imaging in which a series of thin anatomical slices are used to form the three-dimensional structure with help to investigate areas more precisely (Figure 6.15).

6.6.3 ADVANTAGES

Reduces the mortality of women due to breast cancer. Low risk due to low intensity of x-rays is used. In this technique, it also does not require incision, cut, needles, bleeding, or anesthesia. It reduces the risk of the process of chemotherapy as it has side effects.

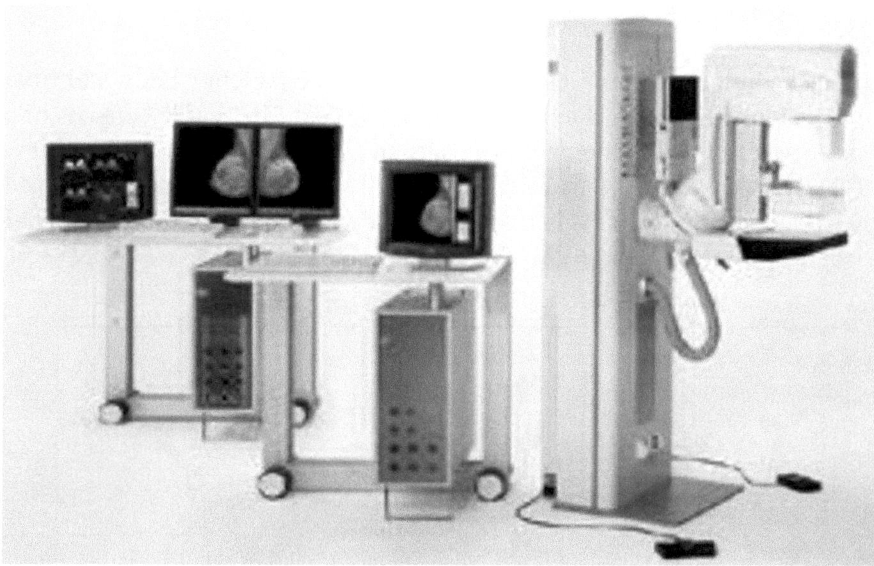

FIGURE 6.15 3D mammography system.

6.6.4 DISADVANTAGES

It requires a skilled and expert operator to examine the affected areas.

6.7 LAPAROSCOPY

Laparoscopy technique is also called keyhole surgery in this technique a small incision is made in the pelvis or abdomen and a long optical fiber cable is used for observing the affected area. Laparoscopy consists of three parts light source, camera unit, and monitor unit. The light source is generally high-intensity halogen or xenon. The camera unit consists of a camera and charge-coupled device which converts the image into electric signals. These electrical signals are then synthesized and obtained in a TV monitor. It is a widely used technique as it provides a real-time image. Hence it has less blood loss, less post-operative pain, avoids shorter hospital stay, early return to normal activity, and minimal risk of incisional hernia.

6.7.1 WORKING

In this technique, a small incision is made on the patient's body and fiber optic cable is placed inside the abdomen. Optical fiber cable consists of a high-resolution camera embedded at its end which provides a wider view of the affected area. In the optical fiber, the high-intensity light is provided by halogen or Xenon. Gas is filled in an abdominal pelvic cavity for better visualization (Figure 6.16).

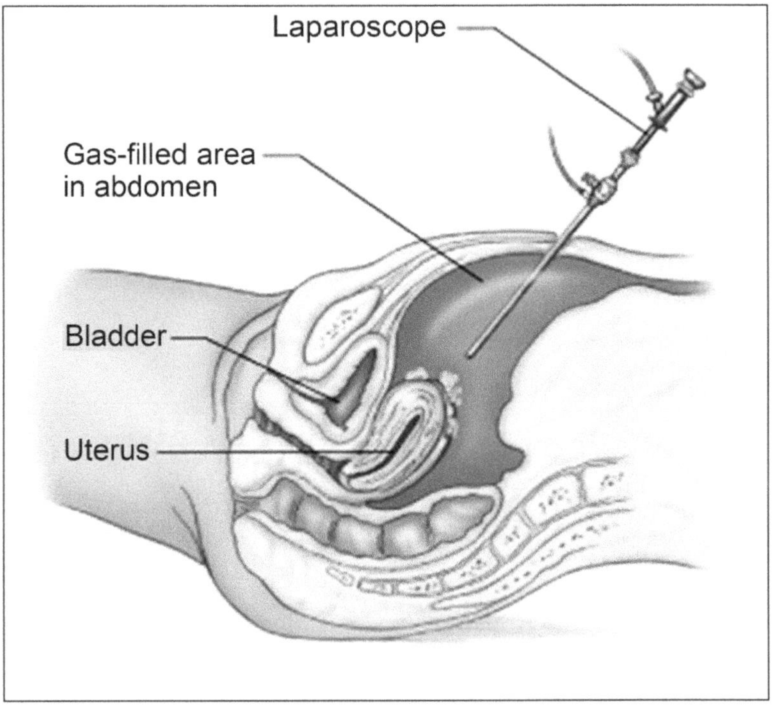

FIGURE 6.16 Laparoscopic system procedure.

The gas used is carbon dioxide as it is rapidly absorbed by the blood. Optical fiber is then maneuvered and moved in all directions to have a panoramic view by the radiologist. The camera consists of a charged coupled device which converts the real-time image into electrical signals. These electrical signals are then synthesized and the image is observed in the TV monitor. The recording is done by a video recorder or DVD recorder.

6.7.2 ADVANTAGES

Laparoscopy is comfortable and is less painful. A small incision takes a small time to heal; therefore, the patient is allowed to get back to his/her regular activities. Laparoscopic surgeries help in reducing the risk of bleeding due to small incision. The amount of blood loss is minimal in such a case and therefore, the need for blood transfusion is also decreased significantly. Another important factor is that, with the help of laparoscopic surgeries, the risk of exposing the internal organs to contamination is also reduced.

6.7.3 DISADVANTAGES

It requires a skilled and expert operator. In this process, there is a chance of complication. This procedure requires the blood bleeding to carry the test. It is case sensitive in case of a person suffering from diabetes and thalassemia in which bleeding does not stop easily.

6.7.4 APPLICATION

It is widely used in the diagnostic of infertility, acute/chronic pelvic pain, ectopic pregnancy, and endometriosis. It is operative in sterilization, ectopic pregnancy, hysterectomy, and tubal anastomoses.

6.8 ELECTROENCEPHALOGRAPHY

Electroencephalography is a technique to track the record of the electrical activity of the brain. In the EEG test, small electrodes shaped like a cup or disc type are placed on the scalp. It records the fluctuation of voltage from the system current to that of neurons of the brain. In this technique, multiple electrodes are placed on the human brain fluctuation of voltage are measured and plotted to measure the electrical activity of the brain in a given time. They pick up the brain's electrical signals and send them to a machine called an electroencephalogram (EEG).

It records the signals on a computer screen or paper. An EEG is mainly used when there is a need to diagnose and manage epilepsy. It can also be used to investigate other conditions such as encephalitis, dementia, head injuries, brain tumors, hemorrhage, and focal brain disorder. It has many advantages low hardware cost, EEG has a very high temporal resolution, in the order of milliseconds rather than seconds. Extremely non-invasive EEG is silent, which allows for better study of the responses to auditory stimuli (Figure 6.17).

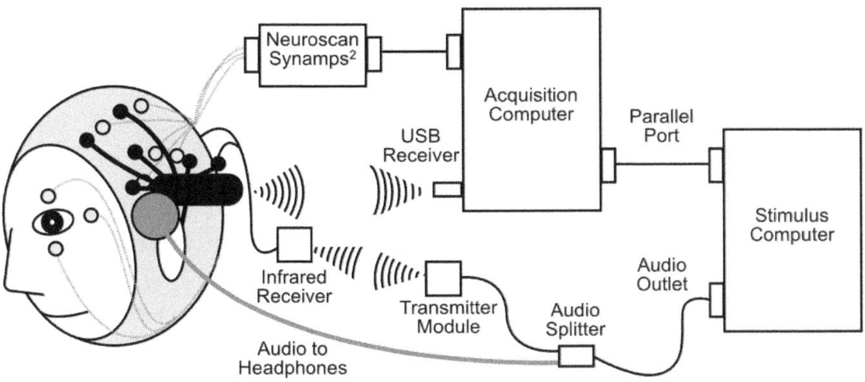

FIGURE 6.17 Electroencephalography system procedure [4].

6.8.1 *WORKING*

In the EEG, electrodes are placed on the brain scalp general the human brain consists of millions of neurons. Neurons continuously exchange ions these ions have the property volume conduction in which ions having the same charge push each other and form a wave when the wave of ions reaches the electrode. Hence electrons are easily capable of attracting and repelling the electron the difference of the acting and repairing voltages are measured and plotted each electrode is connected one input to the difference amplifier and another to the reference electrode. The differential amplifier is the difference in the voltage between the active electrode and the common electrode. The amplified signal then is passed through an anti-aliasing filter then converted to digital by ADC and plotted on the monitor. It records the signals on a computer screen or paper. Many neurological disorders and diseases depend on an accurate assessment of brain function using an EEG [5] (Figure 6.18).

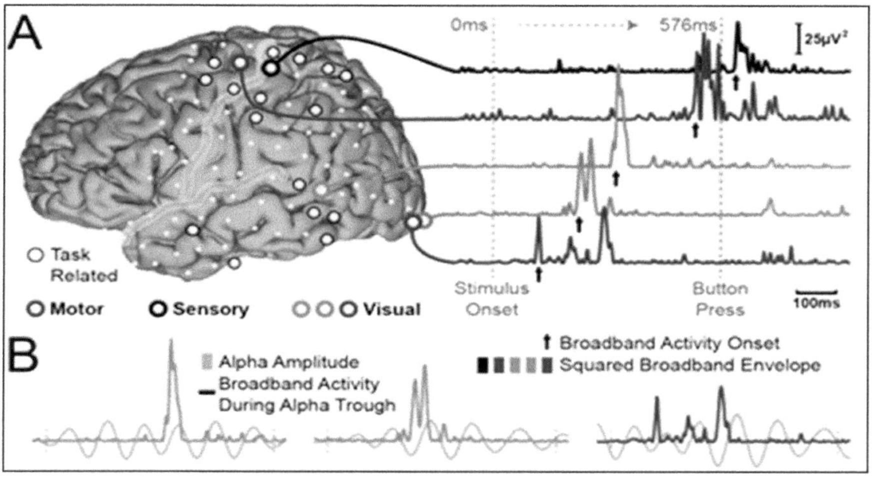

FIGURE 6.18 Two-dimensional voltage plotting according to the electrical activity of the brain net.

6.8.2 ADVANTAGES

It is a non-invasive procedure low risk to the person. It is highly precise, cheap, fast, and accurate in determining the brain activity of the brain. In this technique, it also does not require incision, cut, needles, bleeding, or anesthesia. Hence, it is painless and comfortable to carry out procedures.

6.8.3 DISADVANTAGES

It requires a skilled and expert operator. It has poor spatial resolution and not exact.

6.8.4 APPLICATION

EEG is most commonly used in the diagnosis epilepsy, sleeping disorder, depth of anesthesia, coma, encephalopathies, tumors, brain death, and other focal brain disorders.

6.9 CONCLUSION

Digital image processing and signal image processing have become an integral part of the biomedical diagnostic process due to which accurate diagnostic of element and correct procedure are implemented for any type of disorders or diseases. Also, digital image processing and signal image processing reduces time spent on diagnostic, cost, and reduces the risk of life. Overall, this modern digital image processing and signal image processing are boon to medical practitioners and biomedical engineers also to the suffering patients.

KEYWORDS

- **angiography**
- **Doppler imaging**
- **electroencephalography**
- **laparoscopy**
- **magnetic resonance imaging**
- **mammography**
- **ultrasound**

REFERENCES

1. Dougherty G., (2009). Frontmatter. In: *Digital Image Processing for Medical Applications* (pp. i–iv). Cambridge: Cambridge University Press.
2. Koroshetz, et al., (2018). *Magnetic Resonance Angiography Highlighting the Vasculature in the Human Brain in High Resolution, Without the Use of Any Contrast Agent, on a 7T MRI Scanner*. Courtesy of Plimeni & Wald (MGH). [Note: Here's a great summary on If, How, and When fMRI goes clinical, by Dr. Peter Bandettini.].
3. Evans, D. H., McDicken, W. N., Skidmore, R., & Woodcock, J. P., (1989). *Doppler Ultrasound: Physics, Instrumentation, and Clinical Applications*. Chichester: Wiley.
4. Badcock, N. A., Preece, K. A., De Wit, B., Glenn, K., Fieder, N., Thie, J., & McArthur, G., (2015). Validation of the emotive EPOC EEG system for research quality auditory event-related potentials in children. *Peer J., 3*, e907. https://doi.org/10.7717/peerj.907 (accessed on 29 July 2020).

5. Schalk, G., Marple, J., Knight, R. T., & Coon, W. G., (2017). Instantaneous voltage as an alternative to power and phase-based interpretation of oscillatory brain activity. *NeuroImage, 157*, 545–554. ISSN: 1053-8119.
6. Schalk, G., (2015). A general framework for dynamic cortical function: The function-through-biased oscillations (FBO) hypothesis. *Front Hum. Neurosci., 9,* 352. doi: 10.3389/funhum.2015.00352. eCollection 2015.
7. Craig, F., (2001). *How Ultrasound Works.* HowStuffWorks.com. https://science.howstuffworks.com/ultrasound.htm (accessed on 29 July 2020).
8. Powis, R. L., & Schwartz, R. D., (1991). *Practical Doppler Ultrasound for the Clinician.* Williams and Wilkins.
9. Freudenrich, C., (2001). How ultrasound works. *How Stuff Works*. January 22, 2001.

CHAPTER 7

Finding the Possibility of a Wireless-Based e-Pill for Biomedical Applications

AJAY SHARMA[1] and HANUMAN PRASAD SHUKLA[2]

[1]*Associate Professor, Department of Electronics and Communication Engineering, United College of Engineering and Research, Naini, Prayagraj, Uttar Pradesh–211010, India,*
E-mail: ajaysharma.ucer@gmail.com

[2]*Professor, Department of Electronics and Communication Engineering, United College of Engineering and Research, Naini, Prayagraj, Uttar Pradesh–211010, India,*
E-mail: hpshukla@united.ac.in

ABSTRACT

Whenever we talk about the internal parts of the body or anything that is related with the endoscopy/measurement of the parameters of the inner parts of the body, we always take the approximate data, not the exact data. Can we even think of swallowing any miniaturized PCB, a small digital camera, or any micro digital gadget? Obviously not. We will be scared of doing this. There are a number of constraints in these types of experiments or tests, which start hovering in our minds are health, well-being, and safety. But now, due to the advanced technologies, this has become possible for even human beings. The electronic pills, which are extensively used for the measurement of the internal parameters of the body, are becoming popular and obvious nowadays. They communicate with their base station using the DQPSK technique, even starting at 255 kHz, low carrier modulation. The whole e-pill system can be thought of as consisting of an actuator, which when triggered can deliver the drug inside the stomach/intestines. There will be some electronic circuitry of the transceiver, a battery, few sensors to pick up the temperature, pH of the intestinal fluid, and the SpO_2 level. This arrangement is encapsulated in a body favorable, synthetic material to form a capsule of around 25 mm × 12 mm. Further, there are a number of upgradations that are suggested in the e-pill for better and effective performance and monitoring, which are also discussed later in this chapter.

7.1 INTRODUCTION

If we discuss the latest development of the e-pill (i.e., electronic pill), we will find that in the present communication applications, the accuracy and precision requirements have reached the next level, and a bigger range of full-duplex communication is also required for making it a much systematic and complex integration. Figure 7.1 shows a prototype of the e-pill, finding application in the biomedical field. The pill clearly demonstrates that there are different sections of the e-pill in which various data and parameters are collected and executed for the further use. And if we increase the size of the proposed e-pill to a very small extent, we can measure various other parameters of the inner organs of the body. If we use a high-resolution camera in the e-pill to record all the data and to capture all the pictures of the internal parts of the stomach and intestine, then the data produced by the e-pill will be massive and requires a huge/class storage elements for it. Nowadays the communication is a narrow band, commonly known as the Medical Implant Communication Service (MICS) band, which works on the base frequency of 300 kHz. It has got a range of 1 meter or more based on the type and quality of communication system that has been used in this.

Somewhere in 50's Mackay invented the first of its kind wireless capsule with only one transistor in 1957. And around 1972 the first pH sensor capsule was in reality. Since then research and developments were carried out enhancing and expanding in this field.

The motivation or we can say the objective behind this chapter is that, if anyhow this e-pill succeeds in its aim and objectives, it will be a great panacea for the patients of stomach and intestine, which are suffering from a long time and undergo a painful endoscopy process. And for these, scientists across the world are finding the possibility of a successful e-pill.

The different possibilities of the e-pill, which the researchers took it as a challenge, are explained in chronological order. After 1972, for almost the next 30 years, the researchers kept on practicing on the different modules of the electronic pill, and finally in 2002 "Park" tried an e-pill with a camera sensor of only 510 x 492 pixels, working on 315 MHz. Just two years later, in 2004 "Valdastri" uses a multichannel resolution technology, operating at a basic frequency of 433 MHz, having a data transfer rate of 13 kbps, and uses a regular 3 V coin cell. Just two years later, Johanness tried an e-pill having little lesser data transfer rate of 4 kbps on the same transfer frequency and using the On-Off keying method.

If we can say that all the authors kept on trying for something very effective but didn't succeed fully, so still there is a need for a smart e-pill, with a comparatively higher range, better camera resolution, and an accurate recording of the results.

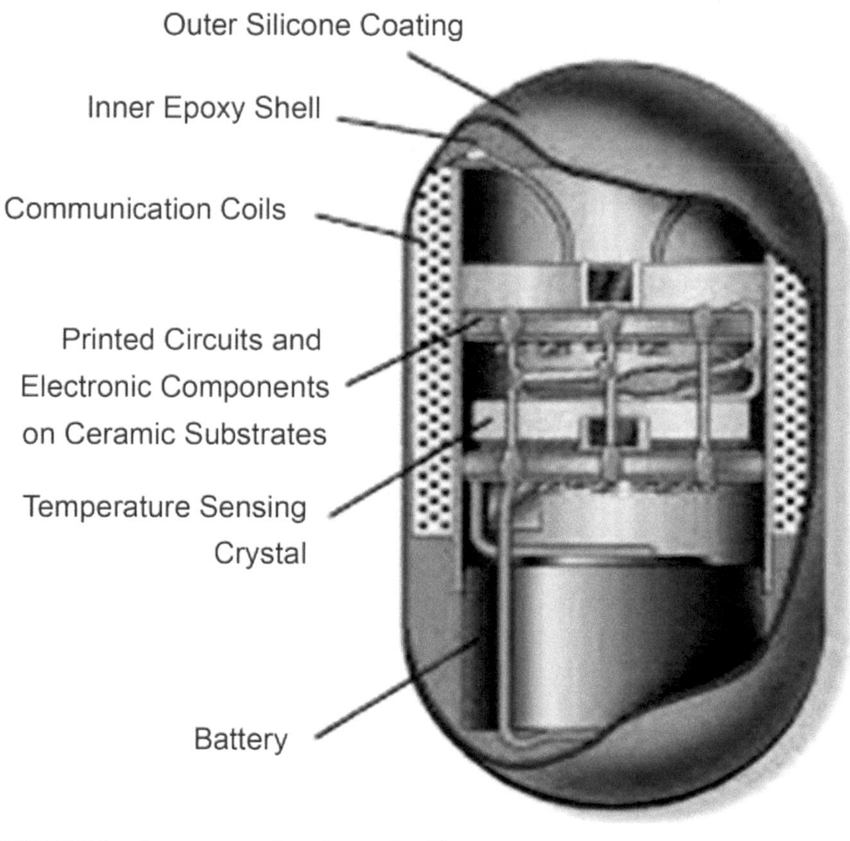

FIGURE 7.1 A prototype of an electronic pill.

7.2 TECHNOLOGY USED IN ELECTRONIC PILL

There has been tremendous growth and researches in this field in order to find out an optimum result in this field and to do a safe recording and measurements of the patients. The efforts started in the world around 1954 and since then, there has been an innumerous advancement in this field of wireless pills, known by different names such as smart capsules, endoradiosondes, wireless pills, smart pill, electronic tablets, etc. The initial attempts were very simple at low frequencies [1, 6]. Hartley and Colpitts oscillator were used initially for this purpose and this topology of connecting a sensor has been used to send the signal from internal parts of the body to external devices. Although being very simple, the early systems were bulky due to large electronic components and the huge batteries used, which use to target temperature, pH, and pressure [8, 9]. As the electronic device should deeply be placed inside the body, which makes the wireless communication interesting due to the medium which has surrounded it, the recent attempts in electronic pills have also been limited to low-frequency transmissions (UHF-433 ISM or lower) [10–16]. Sometimes the low-frequency transmission is really interesting to see, being so accurate and behaving/communicating as per our expectation, with a respectable amount of flexibility. The only disadvantage due to the low frequency is that the electronic components used in the circuit such as capacitors, inductors, etc., are a little larger, making it difficult for realization into an integrated circuit format.

From Table 7.1, it is clearly visible that none of the scientists attempted for any of the frequencies greater than 433 MHz, which means everyone tried to remain from low carrier frequency to the UHF band. Although in the commercial area, there has been extensive use of the larger frequencies for the wireless transmission of the internal vital parameters of the body. One has to be very careful at the higher frequencies due to the ample radiation or the heat emitted from the hardware module of the communication assembly. As in the example given in Ref. [17], the prototype used is with Zigbee compliance, with a very simple and less complex design and occupies an area of $25 \times 14 \times 7$ mm^3. The transmission band which will be used for the medical wireless communication should be unique and pre-allocated in order to avoid interference with other bands. Till the time the so-called electronic pill will not be miniaturized to fit in a capsule of maximum size $30 \times 7 \times 7$ mm^3, it will not be practically feasible in this case.

TABLE 7.1 Recent Facts and Outcomes of the Research Carried Out Across the World on E-Pill

Image Resolution	Image Sensor	Freq.	Data Rate	Modulation	Trans. Power	Physical Dimension	Power Supply	Current Power	References
640 × 480 pixels	MT9V013 (VGA)	144 MHz	2 Mbps	FSK	–18 dBs	Not finalized	3 V coin cell	NA (2 mW for Tx)	[14]
307 × 200 pixels	VGA 0–2 fps	433 MHz	267 kbps	FSK	NA	11.3 × 26.7 Mm × mm	2 × 1.5 V Silver oxide	8 mA (24 mW)	[10]
510 × 480 pixels	PO1200 CMOS	NA	NA	AM	High (variable)	10 × 190 Mm × mm	3 V, wireless	125 mW	[13]
768 × 494 pixels	CCD ICX228AL	UHF	250 kbps	—	NA	20 × 100 Mm × mm	Li-ion battery	—	[16]
510 × 492 pixels	OV7910 CMOS	315 MHZ	NA	AM	NA	10 × 7 Mm × mm	5 V	NA	[15]
pH and Temp. Sensory	pH and Temp.	433 MHz	4 kbps	OOK	NA, 1 m	12 × 36 mm, 8 g	2 × 1.5 V SR48 Ag_2O	15.5 mW	[11]
Multi-channel	Sensors	433 MHz	13 kbps	ASK	5.6 mW 5 m	27 × 19 × 19 mm^3	3-V coin cell (CR1025)	—	[12]
pH, temp., oxygen	Sensors	100 kHz	—	FM	—	—	—	—	[1]

The very next section deals with the practicability of the e-pill and the self-designed model/protocol by the author, which gives a fair idea and detail about the working methodology and the basic operations of the e-pill.

7.3 WIRELESS TELEMETRY AND PRACTICALITY OF THE E-PILL

As we know that the miniaturization is important, different design approaches have been followed by the designers. Figure 7.2 illustrates a proposed prototype of the wireless measurement of the internal parameters of the patient's body, as we can see in the figure, it is clearly depicted that oral e-pill has to be swallowed by the patient. The path traveled by the e-pill is clearly shown in Figure 7.2. As we can see the path of the e-pill is traced and projected side by side or very close to the vital organs of the body, that is, the lever, stomach, and the small intestine. So it takes the exact temperature and pH value of almost all the important parts of the body which is our requirement and objective. The communication system on which we are working is not up to the mark as the range of communication is hardly 1 m or lesser, which needs to be improved. The e-pill also carries high-resolution digital cameras which capture the real-time images and continuously sends at the receiver end which is to be recorded, and by this, we come to know about various diseases, that is, a small cist in the intestine, any wound or internal injury to the patients in case of emergency and accidents [19]. A very small size rechargeable Li-ion batteries were developed especially for this purpose [20]; having a diameter of around 5 mm, shaped in a cylindrical capsule structure. So since then, this prototype is in use.

Figure 7.3 clearly demonstrates the prototype of the drug delivery of the e-pill. As in the figure, it clearly shows that there is a drug reservoir, and after reaching the specific place or position, the actuator is triggered and the fluid pump is activated, resulting in the release of the drug. It is designed to establish a full-duplex communication channel from-to the body, to record temperature or pH value via a temp sensor or chemical sensor. Now we have such type of drug delivery in the smart pills, as we can see that the drug reservoir can be clearly seen in the depicted diagram, and we can also see the drug dispensing hole, in the given capsule, which dispenses the drug on demand when actuated.

In Ref. [13], we see that the robotic endoscope is designed, having a little complex design and is capable of energy transmission as well, making the use of an electromagnetic (EM) coupling. Although in comparison to the other smart devices, this has got a size little bulky and large, it may be due to the extra functions which are proposed to be performed in this e-pill. And this device can be used for a precise drug delivery anywhere in the gastrointestinal (GI) tract of a human being. A recent study in Ref. [14] proposes a prototype using a base data rate frequency of 2 Mbps, for the image resolution to be a little higher. In this, the image resolution can go up to 15 to 20 fps (frames per second) by the use of the available compression techniques such as JPEG, etc. This proposed device is designed to communicate at 144 MHz, comparatively lower than most of the people in this segment, and thus necessitating the use of a larger antenna, which in turn will again increase the size of the pill considerably. Park et al. [15] make the proper use of a simple modulation technique that is AM (amplitude modulation). It incorporates the use of a mixer, an oscillator, a CMOS image sensor, and a loop antenna in its circuitry. And this is one of its kinds of a device which controls the digital capsule inside the human body by an external wireless control unit.

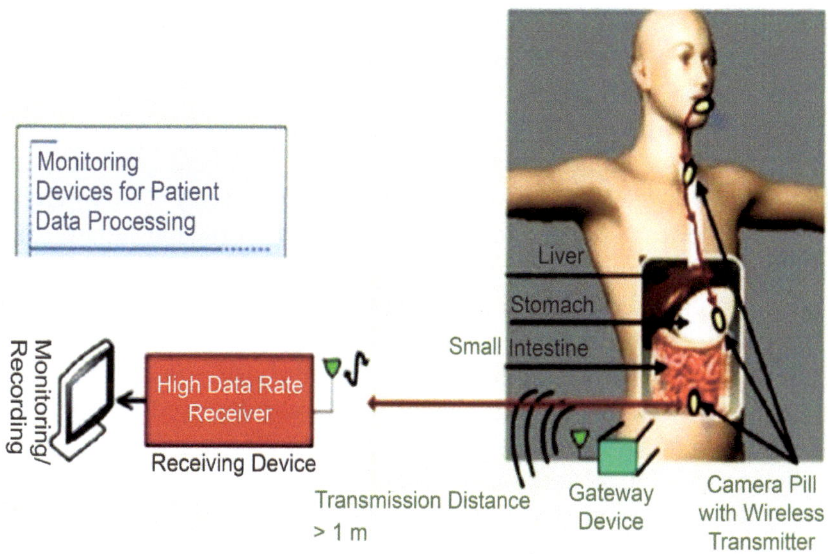

FIGURE 7.2 Wireless telemetry arrangement.

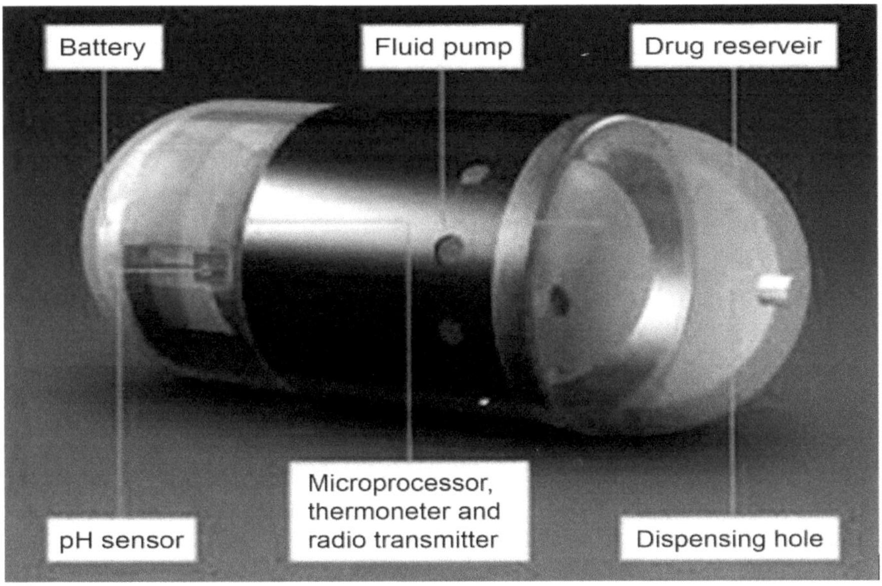

FIGURE 7.3 Prototype of the drug delivery in the e-pill.

Table 7.2 tabulates all types of commercially available e-pills with their exact commercial names and specifications. Among all the PillCam by Given Imaging is the most popular and extensively used e-pill, it is well equipped to diagnose Crohn's disease, cancerous, and benign tumors, celiac disease, ulcerative colitis, Barrett's esophagus, and gastrointestinal reflux disease (GERD) [4]. The endocapsule by Olympus is commercially known as Endocapsule 10, which is widely used for the endoscopy and is capable of taking high-resolution images at a 160-degree wide-angle field of view and provides the visualization of 10% more mucosa as compared to others. It consists of a special mode known as the Omni mode whose smart algorithm removes duplicate and clinically irrelevant images from the data set. Further, the endocapsule can be used as our health monitor, who based on the visual symptoms and signals can suggest to us what to do if it is interfaced with the automatic recorder machine. Now at the third number in Table 7.2, we can find Norika, which is one of the most prestigious projects of the world of developing a battery-free smart pill/microcapsule. The NORIKA system microcapsule is totally powered wirelessly from outside the body. Thus reducing the risk of any toxic substance leakage or dissolution from the batteries. It consists of

TABLE 7.2 Comparison of Different Available Hardware Models from Different Companies

Model	**Company**	**Camera (Sensor)**	**Frequency (MHz)**	**Data Rate**	**Power Source**	**Physical Dimension**	**Image Rate and Resolution**
PillCam (SB)	Given Imaging	Micron, CMOS	402–405 and 433 (Zarlink)	800 kbps (FSK)	Battery	11 × 26 Mm × mm, <4 gr	14 images per second, or 2,600 color images
EndoCapsule	Olympus Optical	CCD camera, 1920 × 1080	—	—	Battery	11 × 26 Mm × mm	2 images per second
Norika	RF System Lab	CCD Image sensor	—	—	Wireless Power	9 × 23 Mm × mm	NA
SmartPill	SmartPill Corporation	Acidity (pH), press, temp.	—	—	Battery	13 × 26 Mm × mm	Only sensor discrete data

a high-quality CCD sensor for the image capturing which is wirelessly powered from outside, and the digital signal processor (DSP) which is supposed to consume maximum power is separated from the internal circuit and is kept outside the body. This capsule can be easily rotated for the detailed examination, which uses the rotation mechanism combining 3-pole motor theory with strobe light effect.

Lastly, the SmartPill motility testing system is manufactured by SmartPill Corporation. This particular pill is capable of measuring pressure, pH, transit time, and temperature as it passes through the intestine of the human being. It can even localize the disease to the specific regions of the tract. We can get the whole gut profile in several minutes; the accuracy of the measurements is incomparable. Although, if it is capable of measuring so many parameters, so the presence of these sensors may give it a bulky look, but removing the battery section from the pill again gives it the same shape and size. Apart from these four commercially available e-pills, there are several newer players in this market, trying hard to make their presence noticeable and few are still on the testing stage for increasing the wireless range of their e-pill. Now in totality, if we take a close look at the above stated four e-pills we conclude that PillcamSB from Given imaging, which has now been taken over by the giant of BioMedical field, Medtronic is the most readily available and economical pill available in the market followed by EndoCapsule.

7.4 CONCLUSION

A lot of work and more efforts are needed to be applied in this topic, and a very high class of transceiver system is required to be incorporated in this, as we want to increase the range of this communication to the max (at least 3 meters). And we have to pay more attention towards the safety of the patients, so that the radiation coming out of this does not put an adverse effect on the body of the patient. Still, much of the research and experiments are being carried out throughout the world on this issue to make it a safe and error-free prototype. Still, much work is required to be done in the exit model of the e-pill after the measurements have been done. Till now only two types of exit module is there, one by the natural bowel motion and the other by tying is a thin plastic thread on the pill and gently pulling it back later, which may result in some mild internal scratches on the internal walls of the tract and stomach. So in the near future, we may also expect a motorized or gliding movement of the e-pill that may also be possible.

KEYWORDS

- **amplitude modulation**
- **digital signal processor**
- **drug**
- **e-pill**
- **gastrointestinal reflux disease**
- **implantable**

REFERENCES

1. Mackay, R. S., (1975). Endpradiossonde. *Nature, 175.*
2. Meron, G., (2000). The development of the swallowable video capsule (M2A). *Gastrointestinal Endoscopy, 6*, 817–819.
3. Meng, M. Q. H., et al., (2004). Wireless robotic capsule endoscopy: State-of-the-art and challenges. In: *The 5th World Congress on Intelligent Control and Automation* (Vol. 6, pp. 5561–5565).
4. Medtronic, (2009). https://www.medtronic.com/covidien/en-us/products/capsule-endoscopy.html (accessed on 29 July 2020).
5. Bradley, P., (2006). An ultra-low-power, high-performance medical implant communication system (MICS) transceiver for implantable devices. In: *The IEEE Biomed. Circuits and Systems Conference* (pp. 158–161).
6. Nagumo, J., et al., (1962). Echo capsule for medical use. *IRE Transaction on Bio-Medical Electronics, 9*, 195–199.
7. McCaffrey, C., et al., (2008). Swallowable-capsule technology. *Pervasive Computing.*
8. Zworykin, V. K., (1957). Radio pill. *Nature, 179*, 898.
9. Mackay, R. S., & Jacobson, B., (1961). Radio telemetering from within the human body. *Science, 134*, 1196–1202.
10. Chen, X., et al., (2009). A wireless capsule endoscope system with low-power controlling and processing ASIC. *IEEE Transactions on Biomedical Circuits and Systems, 3.*
11. Johannessen, E. A., et al., (2006). Biocompatibility of a lab-on-a-pill sensor inartificial gastrointestinal environments. *IEEE Trans. Biomed. Eng., 53*, 2333.

12. Valdastri, P., Menciassi, A., Arena, A., Caccamo, C., & Dario, P., (2004). An implantable telemetry platform system for *in vivo* monitoring of physiological parameters. *IEEE Trans. Inform. Technol. Biomed., 8*, 271.
13. Wang, K., Yan, G., Jiang, P., & Ye, D., (2008). A wireless robotic endoscope for gastro intestine. *IEEE Trans. Robotics, 24*, 206–210.
14. Thone, J., Radiom, S., Turgis, D., Carta, R., Gielen, G., & Puers, R., (2008). Design of a 2 Mbps FSK near-field transmitter for wireless capsule endoscopy. *Sensors and Actuators A: Physical.*
15. Park, H. J., et al., (2002). Design of bi-directional and multi-channel miniaturized telemetry module for wireless endoscopy. In: *Proc. 2nd Int. IEEE-EMBS Conf. Micro Technologies in Medicine and Biology* (pp. 273–276).
16. Kfouri, M., et al., (2008). Toward a miniaturized wireless fluorescence-based diagnostic imaging system. *IEEE J. Selected Topics in Quantum Electronics, 14.*
17. Valdastri, P., Menciassi, A., & Dario, P., (2008). Transmission power requirements for novel Zig Bee implants in the gastrointestinal tract. *IEEE Trans. Biomedical Engineering, 55.*
18. Shin, S. Y., Park, H. S., & Kwon, W. H., (2007). Mutual interference analysis of IEEE 802.15.4 and IEEE 802.11b. *Computer Networks, 51*, 3338–3353.
19. VD6725, (2009). *ST Microelectronics*, http://www.st.com/stonline/products/literature/bd/14370.pdf (accessed on 29 July 2020).
20. Small Battery, (2009). http://www.smallbattery.company.org.uk/hearing_aid_batteries.htm (accessed on 29 July 2020).
21. Jungles, S. L., (2005). Wireless capsule endoscopy a diagnostic tool for early Crohn's disease. *US Gastroenterology Review.*
22. Kim, C., Lehmann, T., Nooshabadi, S., & Nervat, I., (2007). An ultra-wideband transceiver architecture for wireless endoscopes. *International Symp. Communication and Information Tech.*, 1252–1257.
23. Dissanayake, T., Yuce, M. R., & Ho, C. K., (2009). Design and evaluation of a compact antenna for implant-to-air UWB communication. *IEEE Antennas and Wireless Prop. Letters, 8*, 153–156.
24. Aydin, N., Arslan, T., & Cumming, D. R. S., (2005). Design and implementation of a spread spectrum based communication system for an ingestible capsule. *IEEE Trans. Information Technology in Biomedicine, 9.*
25. Murtadha, A., Mehdi, J., & Richard, P. M., (2018). Review of medication adherence monitoring technologies. *Applied System Innovation.* MDPI.

CHAPTER 8

Compact Monopole Antenna with Circularly Polarized Band for Biomedical Applications

SACHIN KUMAR,[1,2] SHOBHIT SAXENA,[3] GARIMA SRIVASTAVA,[4] SANDEEP KUMAR PALANISWAMY,[2] THIPPARAJU RAMA RAO,[2] and BINOD KUMAR KANAUJIA[5]

[1]*School of Electronics Engineering, Kyungpook National University, Daegu–41566, Republic of Korea, E-mail: gupta.sachin0708@gmail.com*

[2]*Department of Electronics and Communication Engineering, SRM Institute of Science and Technology, Chennai–603203, India*

[3]*Department of Electronics Engineering, Indian Institute of Technology (Indian School of Mines), Dhanbad–826004, India*

[4]*Department of Electronics and Communication Engineering, Ambedkar Institute of Advanced Communication Technologies and Research, Delhi–110031, India*

[5]*School of Computational and Integrative Sciences, Jawaharlal Nehru University, New Delhi–110067, India*

ABSTRACT

In this chapter, a new small size antenna with a circularly polarized (CP) band and notched band features are designed. The radiator of the antenna comprises of hexagonal-shaped irregular polygon and a 50 Ω microstrip feeding line. The $S_{11} \geq -10$ dB band of the designed monopole antenna varies from 3.45–5 GHz and 6.6–10.68 GHz with a band elimination notch from 5–6.6 GHz to avoid interference between usable frequency bands. The antenna displays an axial ratio (AR) bandwidth of 200 MHz for 3.5

GHz center frequency. The antenna is simple to fabricate and can be easily incorporated into miniaturized handheld equipments. The antenna overall size is 25×25×1.6 mm^3. The antenna is etched on FR-4 substrate and experimental outcomes are seen in a match with the simulated outcomes.

8.1 INTRODUCTION

Planar monopole antennas are very popular nowadays due to their various advantages, for instance, low profile, low cost, small size, simple fabrication, little power consumption, fast data transmission rate, etc. The major drawback of ordinary microstrip antennas is their small bandwidth, which can be improved by using monopole configuration. In the literature review, it was found that in recent years several shapes like square, rectangular, circular, elliptical, trapezoidal, annular, hexagonal have been proposed for various characteristics of monopole [1, 2]. The resonant bandwidth of the monopole antennas can be enhanced by using different kinds of slots, slits such as circle, rectangle, hexagon, U-and L-shape on the radiating patch or ground surface [3–5]. However, the large bandwidth of the monopole antenna leads to interference between different usable frequency bands. This problem of interference between various application bands can be avoided by designing band-notched monopole antennas. A number of techniques to obtain band rejection characteristics have been proposed by researchers like loading a slot in the patch [6], inserting slits on the patch and ground [7], using stub on the patch [8], conductor backed plane [9], and split-ring resonators (SRR) [10]. Few other methods to create stop band make use of parasitic elements, defected ground structures (DGSs), electromagnetic bandgap (EBG) structures, integrated stop-band filters, and frequency selective surfaces (FSS) above the antennas [11–13].

Circularly polarized (CP) antennas have been popularly used in portable electronic devices for WLAN, WiMAX, GPS, satellite communication, and energy harvesting applications. An ordinary patch antenna radiates radio waves with linear polarization, so misalignment of transceiver antennas can occur. For producing CP waves, two almost equal amplitude orthogonal modes exhibiting a 90° phase change between them are excited simultaneously. A single/dual-feed antenna structure can be used to achieve circular polarization. Single feed antenna exhibits perturbation in the radiating element at an appropriate location for exciting a pair of orthogonal modes exhibiting a 90° phase shift. The antenna structures with dual feed offer broader axial ratio (AR) bandwidth but the main drawback is they need an extra feeding element, which makes antenna geometry complicated. In the last decade, several antenna configurations with one and two feeds have been reported by a lot of people [14–16]. In Ref. [17], a coplanar waveguide (CPW)-fed antenna having asymmetrical ground surface was reported while in Ref. [18], an antenna with simple geometry and asymmetric arm length was designed. Other broadband CP monopole antennas were reported to use the power division system [19], 4 rotated parasitic strips [20], stacked patches [21], etc.

In this chapter, a compact antenna with circular polarization and notched band behavior are presented. The designed microstrip line-fed antenna radiating patch is comprised of an irregular hexagon with slots and slits embedded at the center and periphery. The ground surface of the antenna is a simple modified rectangular plane. The proposed antenna exhibits broadband radiation characteristics with–10 dB impedance bandwidth varying from 3.45–5 GHz and 6.6–10.68 GHz. The antenna covers almost all the useful frequency bands and has an advantage of 200 MHz 3-dB AR bandwidth at 3.5 GHz, thus is capable of radiating CP radiation for the lower WiMAX application band. The electromagnetic (EM) software Ansys HFSS is utilized for carrying out simulation and optimization related to the designed monopole antenna.

8.2 ANTENNA STRUCTURE

Firstly, an irregular polygon with six sides is etched on a substrate of size $25 \times 25 \times 1.6$ mm^3 as illustrated in Figure 8.1(a). This microstrip line-fed design named as antenna-1 resonates from 3.64–10.46 GHz band. Next, a rectangular stub is protruded out from the right side of the antenna with two rectangular slits embedded from the two edges and circular slot-loaded in the asymmetric polygon antenna-1 for achieving circular polarization and band elimination notch between usable bands. The circular slot generates a 90° phase variance among two orthogonal electric field vectors generated by two rectangular slits on the opposite edges of the antenna. Besides this, a rectangular slot of size $l_2 \times W_1$ is etched out from the ground surface to increase gain bandwidth of the antenna structure. The proposed antenna displayed in Figure 8.1(b) resonates from 3.45–5 GHz and 6.6–10.68 GHz with an elimination notch from 5–6.6 GHz to reduce interference between CP WiMAX band and high-speed WLAN (IEEE 802.11a standard).

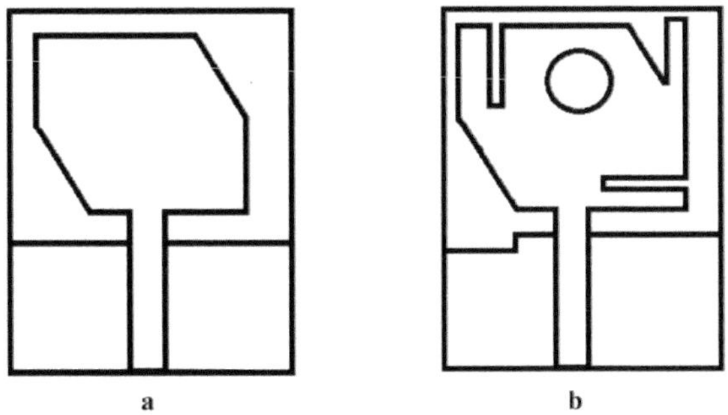

FIGURE 8.1 Design layout of (a) antenna-1 (b) designed antenna.

The design layout details of the antenna are demonstrated in Figure 8.2(a) and antenna dimensional parameters in Table 8.1. The designed antenna is printed on a FR-4 dielectric substrate of 1.6 mm thickness. The picture of the fabricated monopole antenna prototype is displayed in Figure 8.2(b).

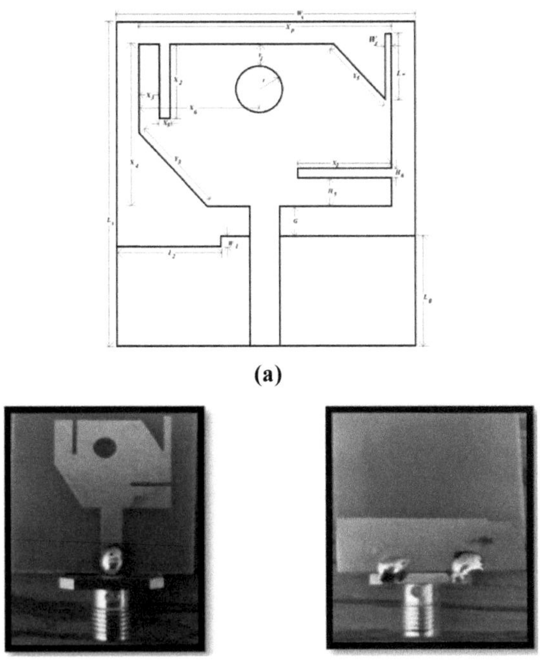

(b)

FIGURE 8.2 Layout of the modified hexagonal antenna (a) design schematic, (b) fabricated prototype.

TABLE 8.1 Dimensional Details of the Proposed Antenna (in mm)

$W_s = 25$	$X_3 = 2.5$	$H_5 = 3.42$	$Y_5 = 6$
$W_4 = 1$	$X_p = 16$	$r = 1.55$	$X_1 = 5.5$
$L_7 = 5.76$	$G = 1.07$	$X_5 = 0.5$	$X_6 = 7$
$H_6 = 0.5$	$L_g = 8.5$	$Y_3 = 8$	
$y_1 = 3.45$	$X_2 = 5.5$	$W_1 = 0.5$	
$L_s = 25$	$X_4 = 13.92$	$l_2 = 4.5$	

8.3 RESULTS DISCUSSION

Figure 8.3 shows the S11 comparison of antenna-1 and the designed antenna. It is found from Figure 8.3 that a band elimination notch from 5–6.6 GHz is achieved in the proposed antenna in comparison with antenna-1. The designed antenna resonates from 3.45–5 GHz and 6.6–10.68 GHz with band elimination notch from 5–6.6 GHz to reduce interference between usable bands. Figure 8.4 displays the AR behavior of antenna-1 and proposed antenna. It is to be noted from Figure 8.4 that a 200 MHz 3-dB AR bandwidth is realized for 3.5 GHz center frequency. The gain comparison of antenna-1 and the proposed antenna is represented in Figure 8.5.

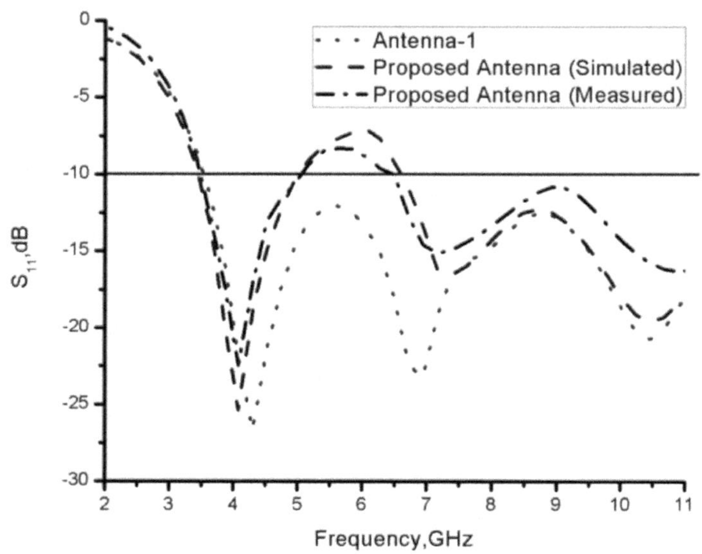

FIGURE 8.3 Reflection coefficient characteristics of antenna-1 and designed antenna.

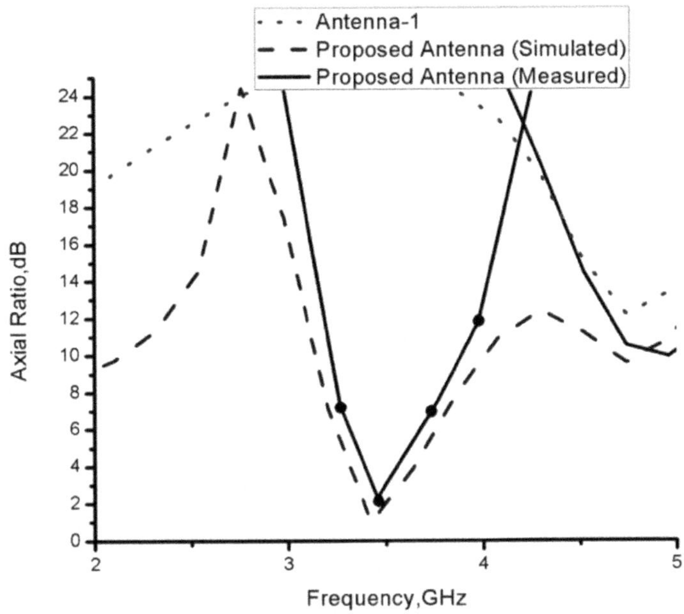

FIGURE 8.4 Axial ratio comparison of antenna-1 and designed antenna.

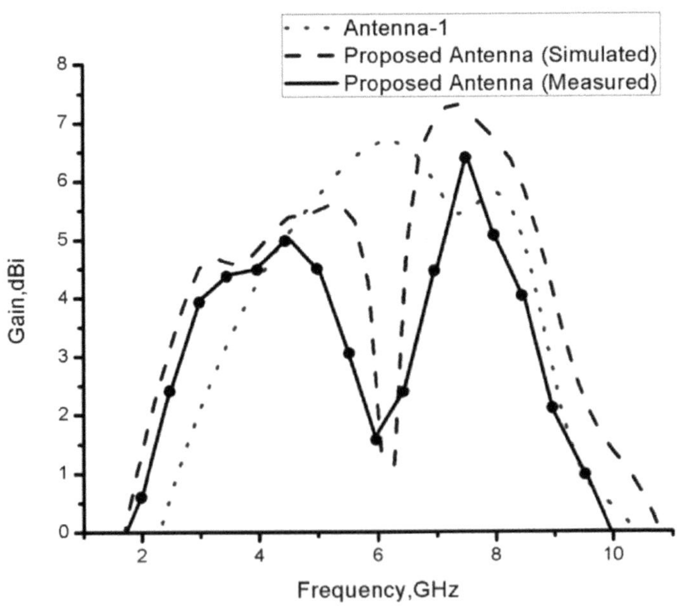

FIGURE 8.5 Gain of antenna-1 and designed antenna.

Figure 8.6 displays the radiation patterns of the antenna. It is noted from the figure that there is a significant difference in right hand circularly polarized (RHCP) and left hand circularly polarized (LHCP) radiation curves. The antenna radiates RHCP waves at 3.5 GHz frequency. Figure 8.7 displays the surface current distribution of the monopole antenna. Figures 8.7(a), (b), (c) and (d) shows the magnitude and resultant direction of current at ωt = 0°, 90°, 180°, and 270°, respectively. It can be seen from the sense of rotation of current that the antenna radiates RHCP waves at 3.5 GHz. The same can be verified from the radiation pattern.

8.3.1 PARAMETRIC STUDY OF THE DESIGNED ANTENNA

In this sub-section, a detailed parametric investigation is presented to illustrate the effect of different parameters used in the designing of the designed configuration. The design factors of the antenna are adjusted on the basis of this parametric study. Figure 8.8 displays S_{11} and AR variation for varying slit length X_2 of the designed antenna. It is seen from Figures 8.8(a) and (b) that the finest value of X_2 is 5.5 mm, which signifies that maximum radiation is achieved at this value. The antenna shows circular polarization radiation only when X_2 is 5.5 mm. The effect of varying slit width X_5 on S_{11} and AR is displayed in Figure 8.9. When the value of X_5 is varied between 0.5 to 1.5 mm, it may be observed in Figure 8.9(a) that the best band-notched characteristic is achieved at 0.5 mm. The effect of the AR at X_5 = 0.5 mm is displayed in Figure 8.9(b).

The varying effects of distance X_3 on S_{11} and AR are shown in Figure 8.10. The X_3 is varied between 1.5 to 3.5 mm and it is observed that the finest value of X_3 is 2.5 mm. At other values of X_3, the band notch bandwidth is small with linear polarization at 3.5 GHz frequency. The effects of the varying radius of circular slot r on S_{11} and AR are displayed in Figures 8.11(a) and (b), respectively. The resonating bands depend on the radius of the circular slot. It is noticed that if the radius of loaded circular slot r is 0.55 mm or 2.55 mm linear polarization radiation is observed while for r =1.55 mm, CP radiation is achieved.

Figure 8.12 displays the effect of distance y_1 on S_{11} and AR of the designed antenna. It is noted from Figure 8.12 that the finest value of y_1 is 3.45 mm. However, at other values of y_1, there is not much significant

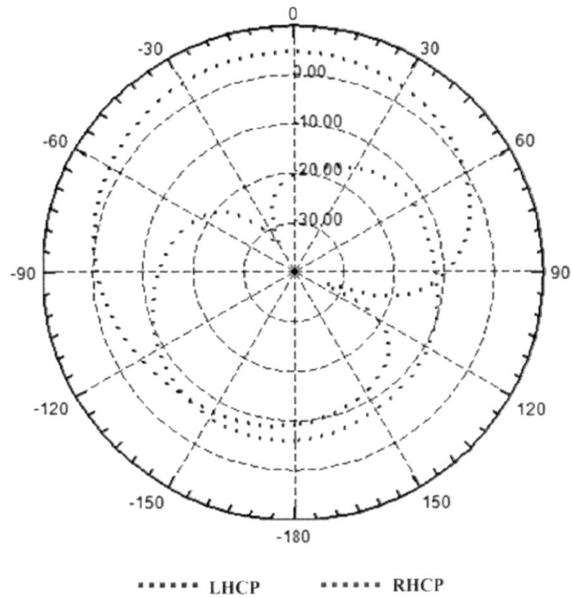

(a)

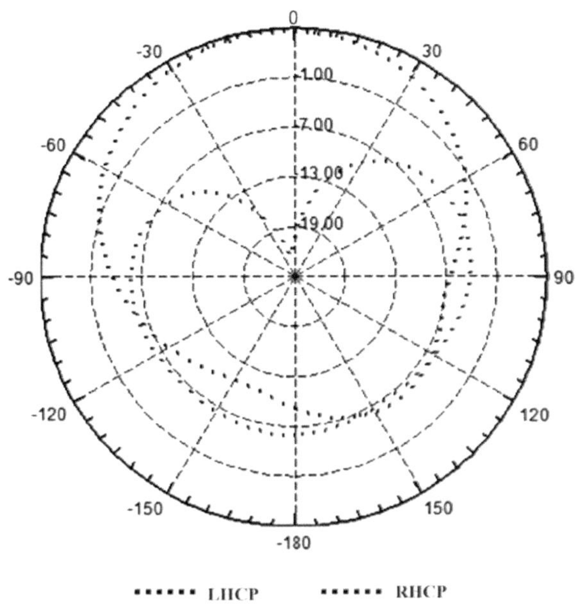

(b)

FIGURE 8.6 Radiation patterns of the designed antenna at 3.5 GHz (a) $\varphi = 0°$ (b) $\varphi = 90°$.

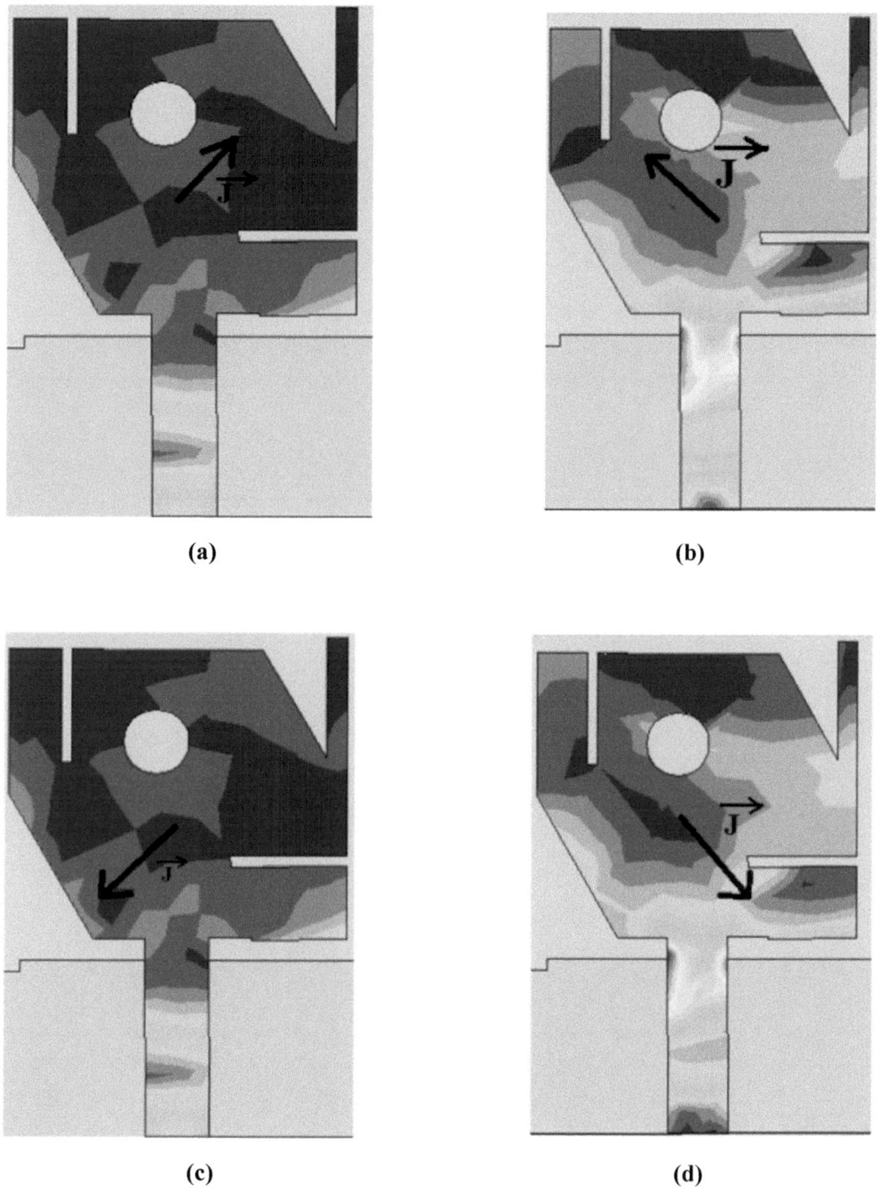

FIGURE 8.7 Magnitude of surface current at 3.5 GHz at (a) $\omega t = 0°$, (b) $\omega t = 90°$, (c) $\omega t = 180°$, and (d) $\omega t = 270°$.

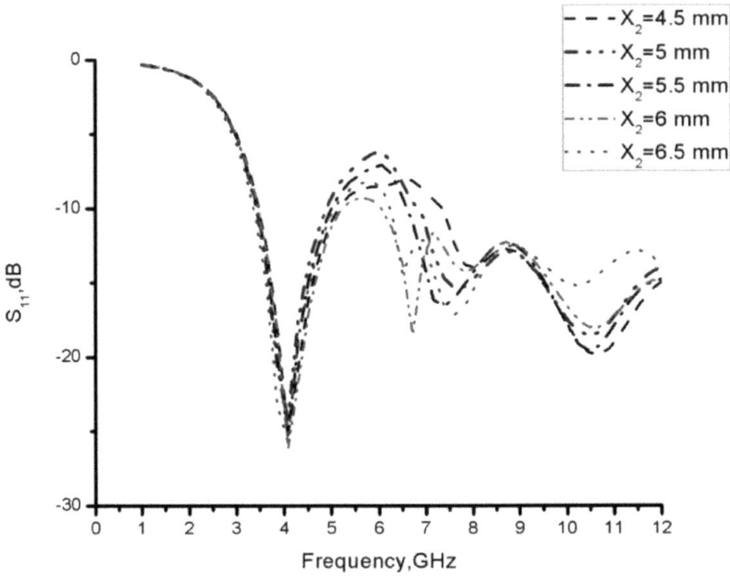

(a)

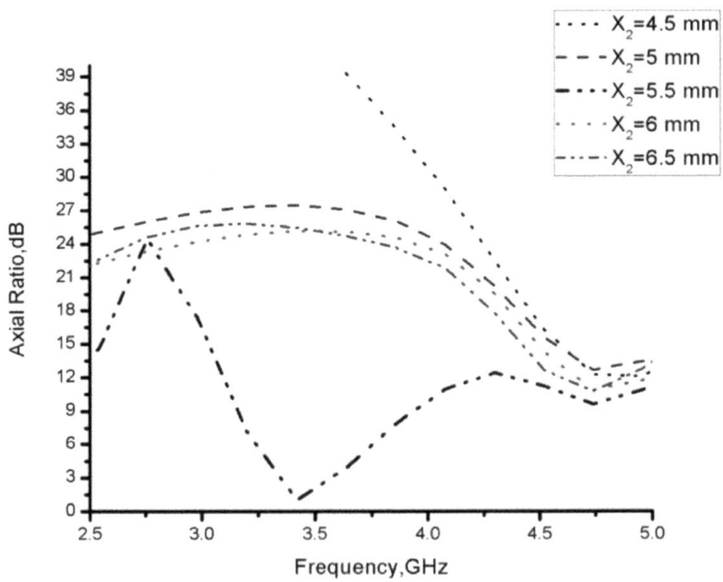

(b)

FIGURE 8.8 Frequency variation for different values of X_2 (a) S_{11} (b) axial ratio.

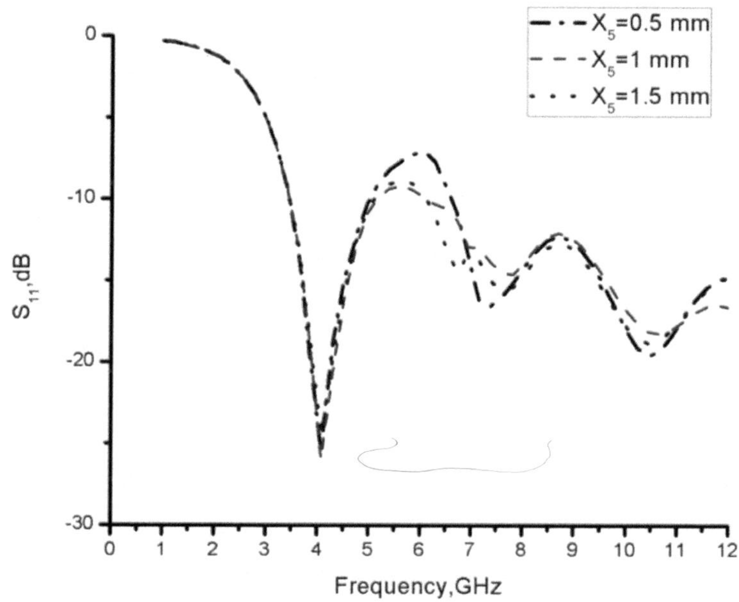

(a)

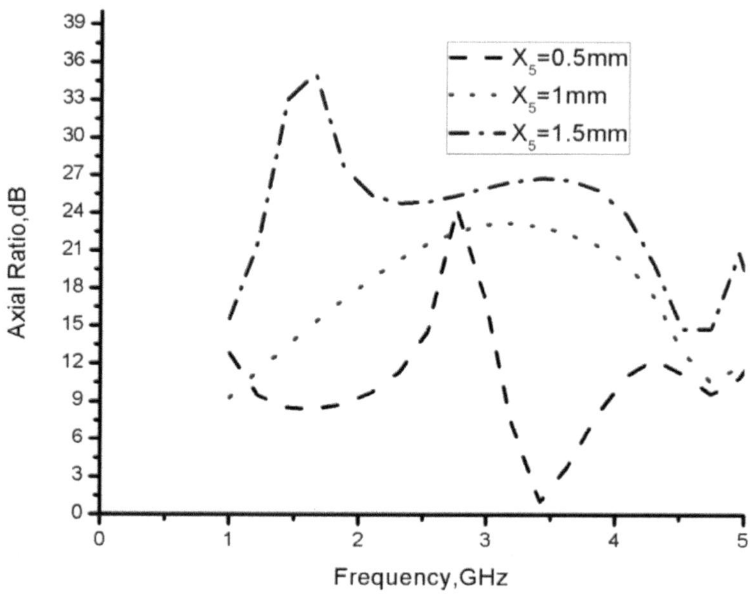

(b)

FIGURE 8.9 Frequency variation for different values of X_5 (a) S_{11} (b) axial ratio.

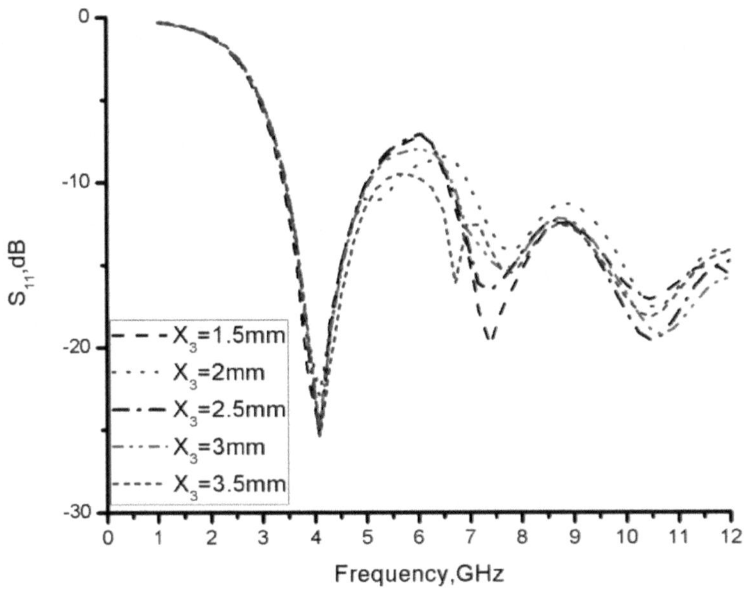

(a)

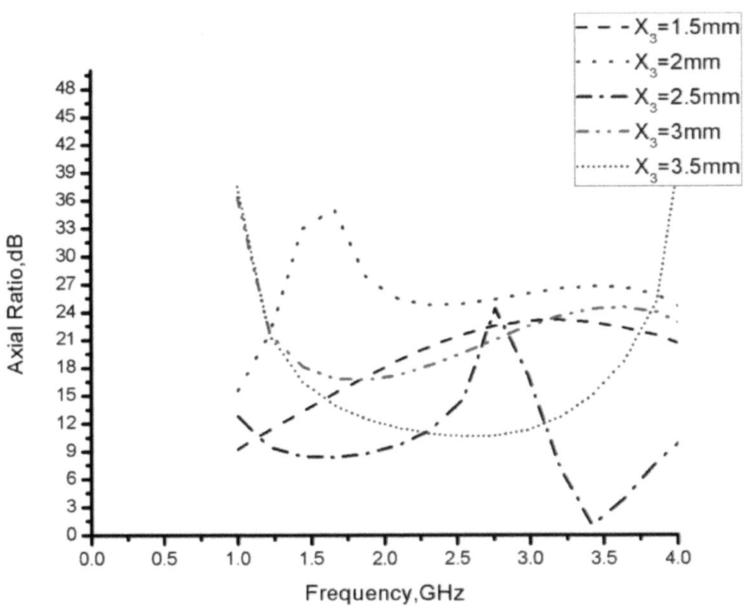

(b)

FIGURE 8.10 Frequency variation for different values of X_3 (a) S_{11} (b) axial ratio.

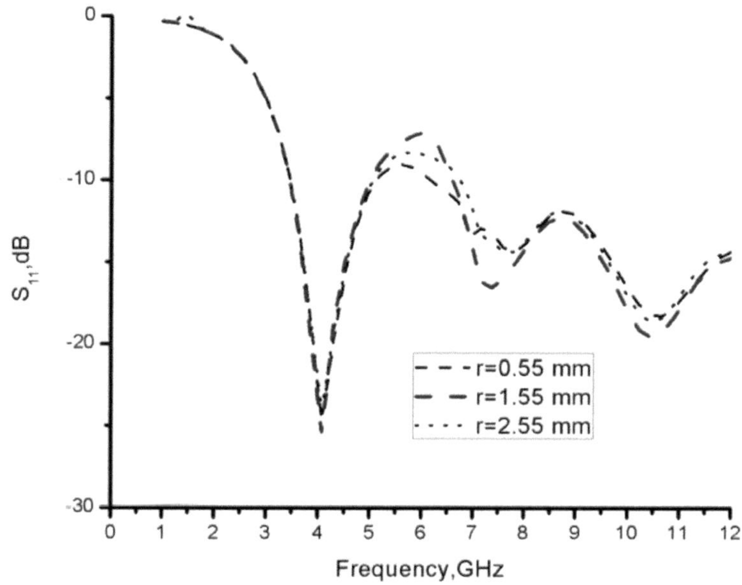

(a)

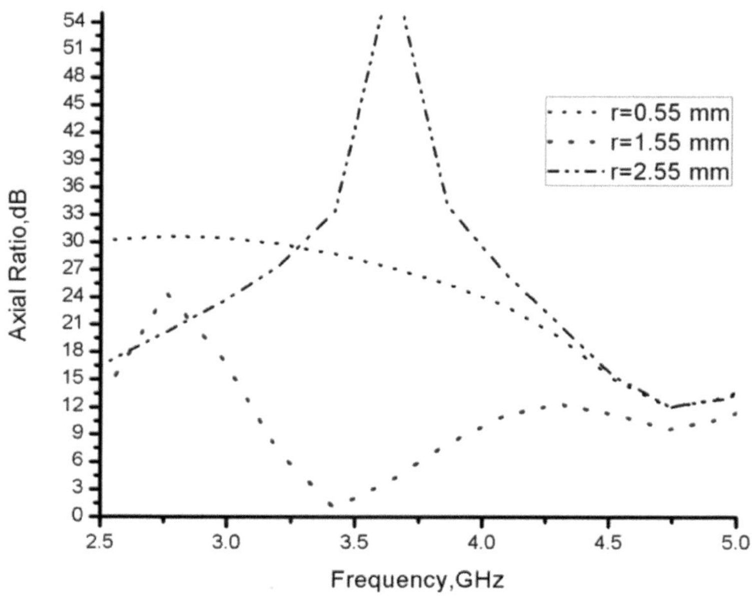

(b)

FIGURE 8.11 Frequency variation for different values of *r* (a) S_{11} (b) axial ratio.

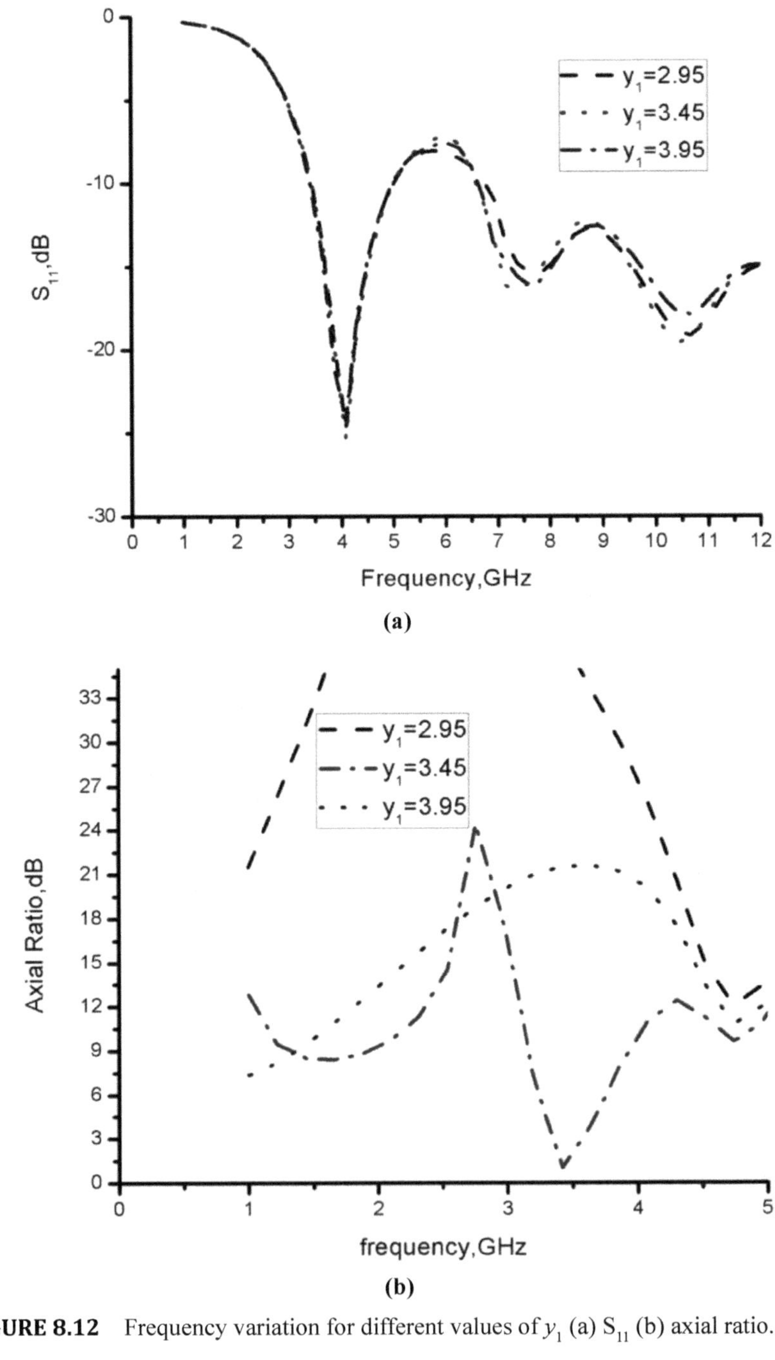

FIGURE 8.12 Frequency variation for different values of y_1 (a) S_{11} (b) axial ratio.

difference in the return loss but the radiation polarization varies. The effects of varying slit length X_1 on S_{11} and AR are shown in Figure 8.13. The length differs from 4.5 to 6.5 mm and is seen that at a smaller value of X_1 the notch is not present in the S_{11} graph and the antenna exhibits linearly polarization radiation, while for high values of X_1 the notch bandwidth is enhanced. It is noticed from the figure that the finest value of X_1 is 5.5 mm.

The effects of varying width H_6 on S_{11} and AR of the designed antenna are presented in Figures 8.14(a) and 8.14(b), respectively. It is understood from Figure 8.14(a) that there is not much significant difference in return loss bandwidth for different H_6 values while the AR is achieved only when H_6 is 0.5 mm. Figure 8.15 depicts the outcome of altering distance H_5 on S_{11} and AR of the antenna. The notch bandwidth of the antenna falls by enhancing the length H_5. The AR and frequency deviation for different H_5 is represented in Figure 8.15(b) and it is found that the AR is achieved only when H_5 is 3.42 mm.

Figure 8.16 shows the effect of varying stub L_7 on S_{11} and AR of the designed antenna. There is a lot of variation in notch bandwidth for different L_7 values. At lower values of L_7, the notch is not present in the return loss range while for higher values the bandwidth of notch is small. It can be observed from Figures 8.16(a) and (b) that the finest value of L_7 is 5.76 mm. The effect of varying stub width W_4 on S_{11} and AR is displayed in Figures 8.17(a) and (b). And it is found from the figure that the best value of W_4 is 1 mm. For lower W_4 values, the antenna does not radiate to a large amount with a shift in notch band. Also, the radiation is linear at high stub width.

8.4 CONCLUSION

In this chapter, a new small size antenna is designed for wideband applications with an added advantage of the CP band at 3.5 GHz. The antenna resonates from 3.45–5 GHz and 6.6–10.68 GHz with an elimination notch from 5–6.6 GHz to reduce interference between CP WiMAX band and high-speed WLAN (IEEE 802.11a standard). The designed monopole antenna can be simply integrated with other high-frequency devices or microwave equipments.

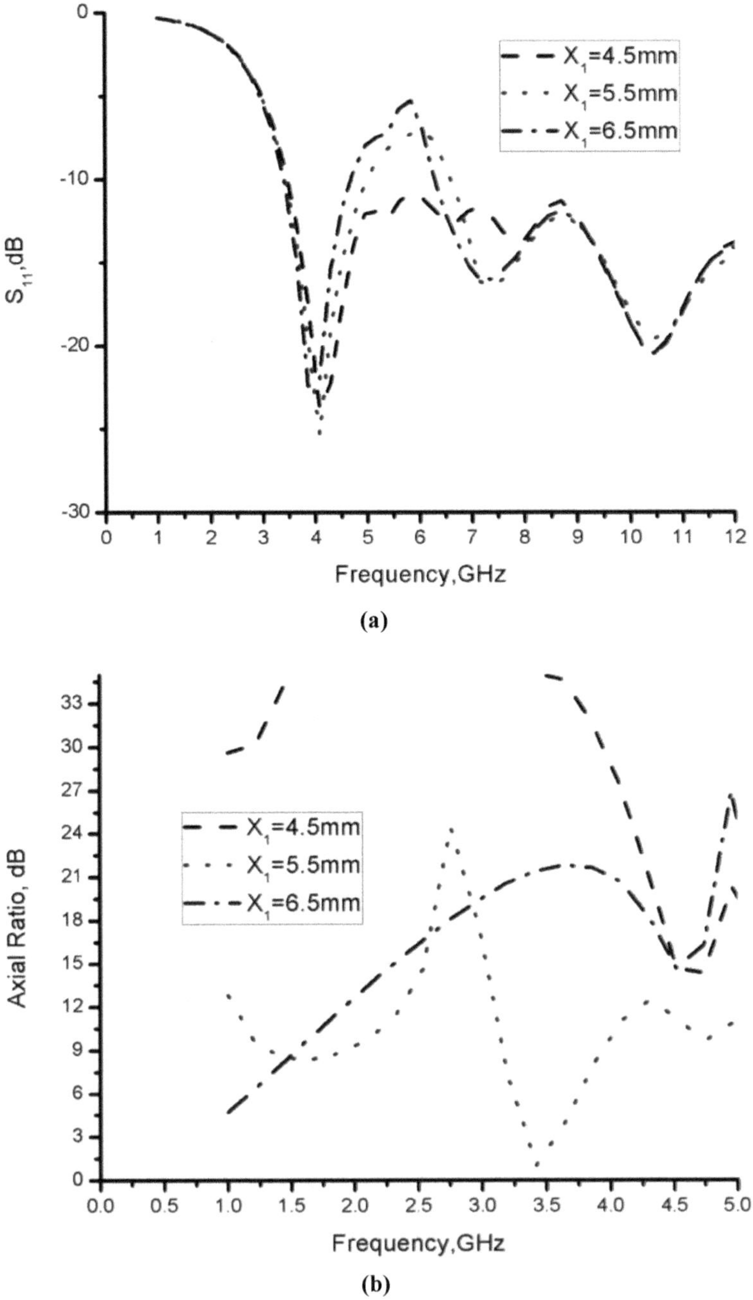

FIGURE 8.13 Frequency variation for different values of X_1 (a) S_{11} (b) axial ratio.

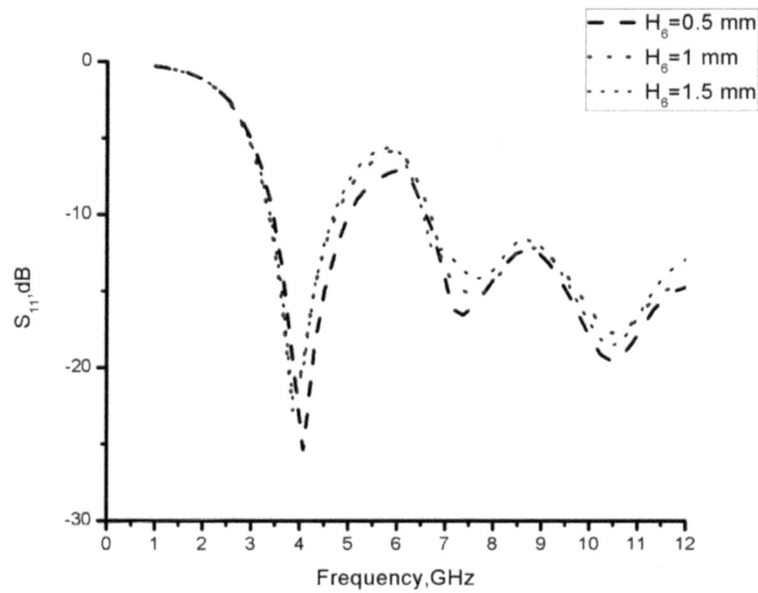

(a)

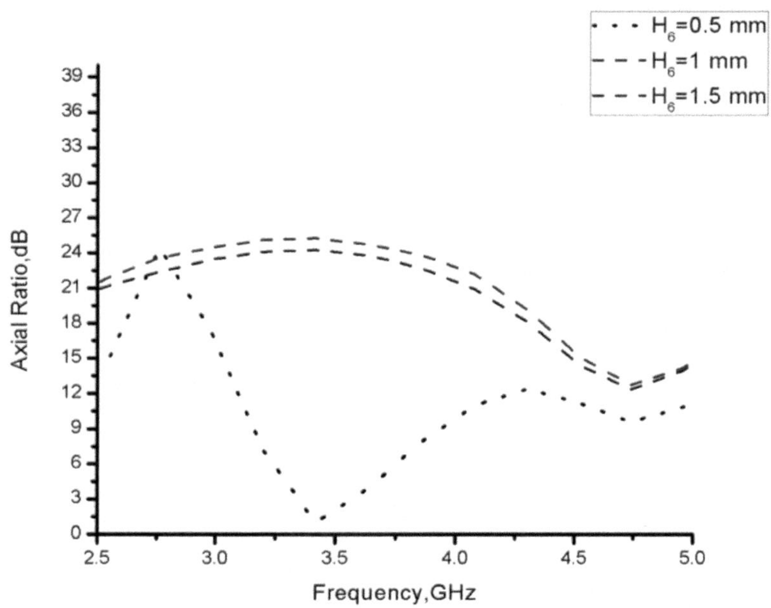

(b)

FIGURE 8.14 Frequency variation for different values of H_6 (a) S_{11} (b) axial ratio.

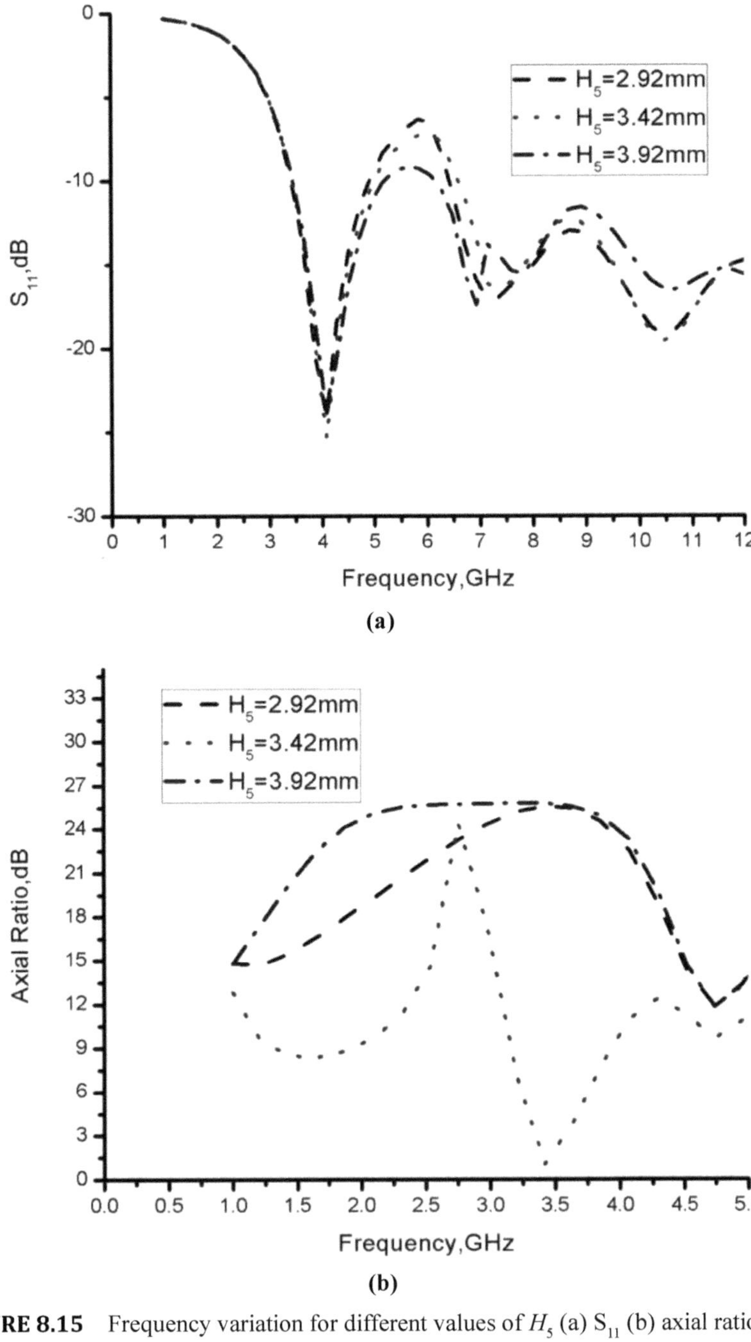

FIGURE 8.15 Frequency variation for different values of H_5 (a) S_{11} (b) axial ratio.

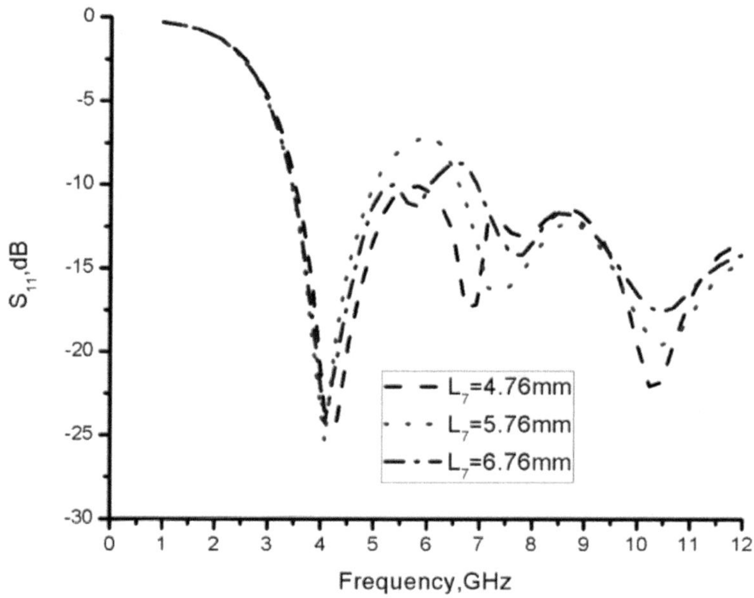

(a)

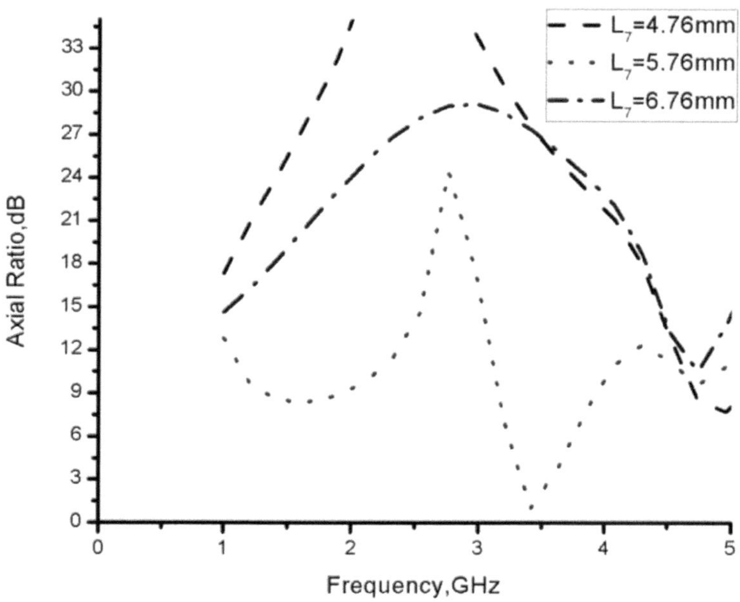

(b)

FIGURE 8.16 Frequency variation for different values of L_7 (a) S_{11} (b) axial ratio.

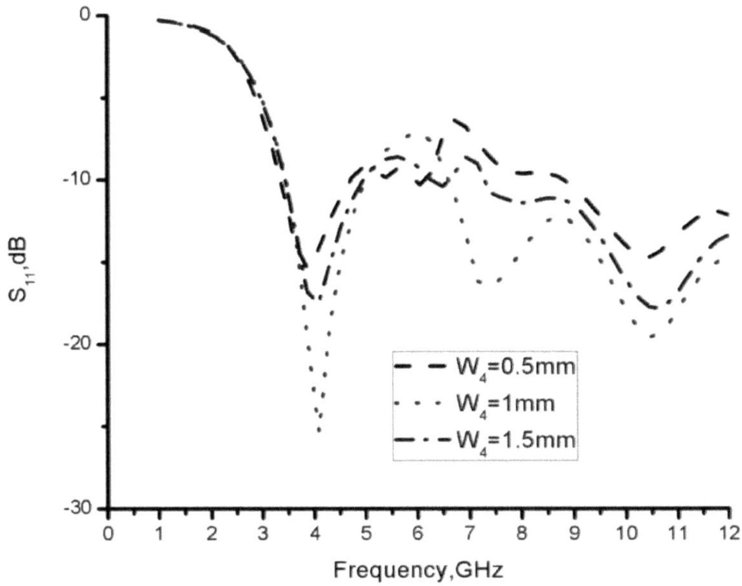

(a)

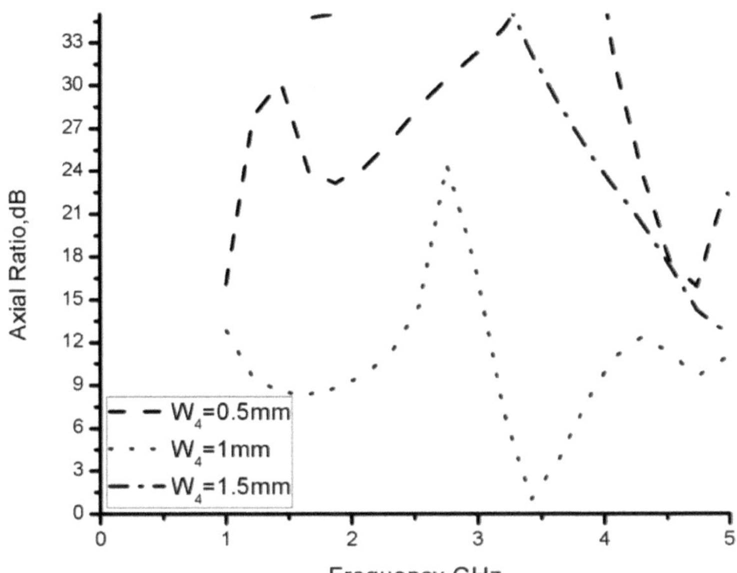

(b)

FIGURE 8.17 Frequency variation for different values of W_4 (a) S_{11} (b) axial ratio.

KEYWORDS

- **antenna**
- **coplanar waveguide**
- **electromagnetic bandgap**
- **frequency selective surfaces**
- **monopole**
- **notch**

REFERENCES

1. Chen, Z. N., Ammann, M. J., Qing, X. M., Wu, X. H., See, T. S. P., & Cai, A., (2006). Planar antennas. *IEEE Microw. Mag., 7*, 63–73.
2. Bakariya, P. S., Dwari, S., Sarkar, M., & Mandal, M. K., (2015). Proximity-coupled multiband microstrip antenna for wireless applications. *IEEE Antennas Wireless Propag. Lett., 14*, 646–649.
3. Bakariya, P. S., Dwari, S., Sarkar, M., & Mandal, M. K., (2015). Proximity-coupled microstrip antenna for Bluetooth, WiMAX, and WLAN applications. *IEEE Antennas Wireless Propag. Lett., 14*, 755–758.
4. Khandelwal, M. K., Kanaujia, B. K., Dwari, S., Kumar, S., & Gautam, A. K., (2014). Bandwidth enhancement and cross-polarization suppression in ultra-wideband microstrip antenna with defected ground plane. *Microw. Opt. Technol. Lett., 56*, 2141–2146.
5. Bhatia, S. S., & Sivia, J. S., (2016). A novel design of circular monopole antenna for wireless applications. *Wireless Per. Commun., 91*, 1153–1161.
6. Fallahi, R., Kalteh, A., & Roozbahani, M., (2008). A novel UWB elliptical slot antenna with band-notched characteristics. *Progress in Electromagnetics Research, 82*, 127–136.
7. Sim, C. Y. D., Chung, W. T., & Lee, C. H., (2008). Novel band-notch UWB antenna design with slit ground plane. *Microw. Opt. Technol. Lett., 50*, 2229–2233.
8. Koohestani, M., & Golpour, M., (2010). U-shaped microstrip patch antenna with novel parasitic tuning stubs for ultra-wideband applications. *IET Microw. Antennas Propag., 4*, 938–946.
9. Moradhesari, A., Moosazadeh, M., & Esmati, Z., (2012). Band-notched UWB planar monopole antenna using slotted conductor-backed plane. *Microw. Opt. Technol. Lett., 54*, 2237–2241.
10. Siddiqui, J. Y., Saha, C., & Antar, Y. M. M., (2014). Compact SRR loaded UWB circular monopole antenna with frequency notch characteristics. *IEEE Trans. Antennas Propag., 62*, 4015–4020.

11. Zaker, R., Ghobadi, C., & Nourinia, J., (2008). Novel modified UWB planar monopole antenna with variable frequency band-notch function. *IEEE Antennas Wireless Propag. Lett.*, *7*, 112–114.
12. Hong, C. Y., Ling, C. W., Tarn, I. Y., & Chung, S. J., (2007). Design of a planar ultrawideband antenna with a new band-notch structure. *IEEE Trans. Antennas Propag.*, *55*, 3391–3396.
13. Kim, K. H., Cho, Y. J., Hwang, S. H., & Park, S. O., (2005). Band-notched UWB planar monopole antenna with two parasitic patches. *Electron. Lett.*, *41*, 783–785.
14. Saxena, S., Kanaujia, B. K., Dwari, S., Kumar, S., & Tiwari, R., (2017). A compact microstrip fed dual-polarized multiband antenna for IEEE 802.11 a/b/g/n/ac/ax applications. *AEU-Int. J. Electron. Commun.*, *72*, 95–103.
15. Cao, W., Zhang, B., Yu, T., & Li, H., (2010). A single-feed broadband circular polarized rectangular microstrip antenna with chip-resistor loading. *IEEE Antennas Wireless Propag. Lett.*, *9*, 1065–1068.
16. Kanaujia, B. K., Kumar, S., Khandelwal, M. K., & Gautam, A. K., (2015). Single feed L-slot microstrip antenna for circular polarization. *Wireless Per. Commun.*, *85*, 2041–2054.
17. Wang, C. J., & Hisao, K. L., (2014). CPW-fed monopole antenna for multiple system integration. *IEEE Trans. Antennas Propag.*, *62*, 1007–1011.
18. Ghobadi, A., & Dehmollaian, M., (2012). A printed circularly polarized Y-shaped monopole antenna. *IEEE Antennas Wireless Propag. Lett.*, *11*, 22–25.
19. Kumar, T., & Harish, A. R., (2013). Broadband circularly polarized printed slot-monopole antenna. *IEEE Antennas Wireless Propag. Lett.*, *12*, 1531–1534.
20. Wu, J., Yin, Y., & Wang, Z., (2015). Broadband circularly polarized patch antenna with parasitic strips. *IEEE Antennas Wireless Propag. Lett.*, *14*, 599–602.
21. Kumar, S., Kanaujia, B. K., Khandelwal, M. K., & Gautam, A. K., (2014). Stacked dual-band circularly polarized microstrip antenna with small frequency ratio. *Microw. Opt. Technol. Lett.*, *56*, 1933–1937.

CHAPTER 9

Machine Learning Implementations in Bioinformatics and Its Application

SHIKHAR SHARMA and MANJU KHARI

Ambedkar Institute of Advanced Communication Technologies and Research, Geeta Colony, Delhi–110031, India,
E-mail: manjukhari@yahoo.co.in (M. Khari)

ABSTRACT

This chapter is based on the implementation of machine learning (ML) methods in biomedical science. It is also termed as bioinformatics as there are dealings with huge chunks of data in the biomedical field. Since there is a drastic increase in data of biomedical science analysis and predictions using ML is quite beneficial. In biomedical research predictions of diseases, classification of the type of disease, and insights based on data provided can help humanity and society a lot. In this chapter, it has been studied classification techniques with background and functioning of supervised ML models such as decision tree (DT), support vector machines (SVMs), and K-nearest neighbor and their implementation on breast cancer dataset. ML methods create a healthcare chatbot system that can provide a possible prediction of disease based on symptoms asked by a chatbot.

9.1 INTRODUCTION

Machine learning (ML) is about the abstraction of data and having predictive analysis on that data. The term ML was coined by Samuel of Stanford University in 1959 [1]. According to him, ML is the art and science of training machines without being explicitly programmed. A more engineering-oriented definition of ML was given in Ref. [2]. The definition states that a machine is said to have learned with experience 'E' on some task 'T' with a performance measure 'P,' if on task 'T' the performance measure 'P' increases with experience 'E.' ML is an old branch of study but its application has increased tremendously in recent times due to an exponential increase in the amount of data available and the performance of computers to handle such a huge amount of data has also increased. Its application is not limited to the computer science field rather it expands in every domain and sectors wherever there is a need to have predictive or statistical analysis.

ML applications or models generally comprise of a particular procedure that includes extraction of data, making data readable to the computer system, that is, data preprocessing, after preprocessing data it is visualized for finding out different trends or important features. This whole process till visualization can be clubbed into data analysis which is a further detailed study branch. After whole preprocessing and analysis of data, it is necessary to find which type of ML algorithms could be applied to data, after successful testing and tuning of the algorithm on data, and after having acceptable results, the model can be deployed.

In the field of biomedical science, ML can play a vital role in the research and healthcare sector [3]. It can have very vast applications such as predictions of diseases with symptoms data provided, classification different body conditions, and disease with image analysis, DNA sequence analysis, and much more. Most of the real-world data in the biomedical field consist of huge amounts of data this data can be studied using ML and deep learning methods to find relevant information and results which can be difficult for manual study [21, 22]. With such increment in data in the biomedical field, there a separate branch of studies has evolved known as bioinformatics [4]. This chapter is made with the motivation for the study of ML in biomedical science and applying relevant data for results.

In this chapter, the first pre-concepts of ML are discussed and there is a discussion related to the preprocessing of data, after that background and working of different ML algorithms are discussed, their case study, and results on the breast cancer dataset are studied. At last, the best ML algorithms have been applied to create a healthcare chatbot system where a series of questions are asked to users related to symptoms given and disease is predicted with a link to a doctor related to that disease is provided to the user. In the conclusion of this chapter, aspects of health care chatbot and the future scope of ML and deep learning techniques in the biomedical field are discussed.

9.2 MACHINE LEARNING (ML) PRE-CONCEPTS

ML is a branch of study where both input and output to the computer are provided and the computer system tries to find the patterns relations and trends in that data using statistical and probabilistic methods. Problems in ML could be regression-based or classification based, wherein regression-based problems data tends to follow a linear or curve nature. But most of the problems are classification based where there is a need to classify data into different classes [5, 6]. Classification could be binary where only two classes are present or *n*-ary, where there are *n* number of classes are possible. But there are few more ways to classify of a ML model or application which are the following:

1. Whether or not the ML system needs human supervision.
   - Supervised learning is when data is labeled, that is, particular results are already provided and the system is trained to find results based on previous results when new data is provided.
   - Unsupervised learning is when data in an unlabeled here system tries to find out different trends and insights from data [7].
   - Semi-supervised learning is when consists of both labeled and unlabeled observations [8].
   - Reinforcement learning is when the system tries to learn from previous mistakes and it tries to find the best possible decisions or behavior it should take in a particular situation [9]
2. Whether or not the ML system can incrementally learn on the fly.
   - Online learning is when the system tries to find prediction on every new set of observations, that is, the model is updated on every new set of observations in sequential order.
   - Batch learning is when a model finds out results after learning from the whole dataset and not at every step of observation.
3. Whether the ML system generalizes on a known set of points or rather creates a model.
   - Instance-based learning is when the system makes all processes of prediction making for every new instance or feature; hence, all steps are repeated for every new feature [10].
   - Model-based learning is when a system makes a model based on all features provided and once a model is created, it tries to find a prediction for any new set of features based on the model generated [11].

In this chapter, there is the main focus on supervised learning where data with both inputs and results are provided to the ML algorithm, and when a new set of values in input are provided algorithm predicts output according to the relation it derives by analysis data given above. In a supervised ML model or application, in the dataset, there are the following terms defined as X = feature matrix, y = vector of observations, m = number of observations, x = dataset, and n = number of features. All the operations are performed on the data set are done considering X as features that will result in prediction y. Now the dataset has to be defined into X and y, ML algorithm will be applied on the whole data set and when will provide new set values of features given will be provided, a prediction is made.

Data preprocessing is a crucial step in the ML and data mining processes and models. Methods of gathering the data are often lightly controlled which results in outlying values, impossible data combinations, missing values, etc. [12]. Data which is analyzed without proper preprocessing could lead to misleading results. Thus, the representation and quality of data should be very important before running an analysis. Data preprocessing is the most important phase of a ML project, especially in computational biology. Training of ML models with irrelevant redundant noisy data could result in unwanted outcomes. Data preparation and filtering steps can take a considerable amount of processing time. Before the application of algorithms, data is needed to be preprocessed accordingly where the model should be tackled with categorical data, missing values, dummy variable trap, and scaling of whole data. For all the abovementioned problems, the sci-kit learns the library of python has been used for data preprocessing and ML algorithms.

In the next section, the background and working of the different classification algorithms are discussed, where brief information about the different algorithms is discussed and the working of a major ML algorithm is provided.

9.3 BACKGROUND AND WORKING OF MACHINE LEARNING (ML) ALGORITHMS

ML model or system works by using different algorithms, which are studied thoroughly in the past. These algorithms help in finding results in different problems. Majorly all algorithms are classified into two types classification and regression-based algorithms as discussed in the above section. In classification algorithms, they can further be classified into a probabilistic and deterministic algorithm. Probabilistic algorithms are those which give a probability of classification results, that is, when giving results these algorithms provide the probability of a particular instance of being in a class, a class with the highest probability is given as a result of that particular instance. In contrast, deterministic algorithms are those where results are given with 100% surety that a particular instance belongs to that particular class. In this chapter, three main deterministic algorithms are discussed that are decision tree (DT), support vector machine (SVM), and K-nearest neighbors.

9.3.1 DECISION TREE (DT)

The decision tree (DT) algorithm is a deterministic model-based technique that is suitable for n-ary classification problems [13]. It is suitable for moderately large datasets. The DT algorithm tries to fit the whole dataset in a tree structure where every node represents an attribute and through a series of if-else questions, it finally has child nodes as a prediction of a particular classification. The DT algorithm uses some measure of impurity to create an optimal split. The most preferred of which are the Gini Index and Entropy (or Information Gain). Based on some measure of impurity, the DT algorithm attempts to minimize the cost function, represented by J, calculated for every pair of (k, t_k). The DT algorithm chooses some measurement of impurity to create an optimal split based on one of the following two methods:

1. Gini index or Gini impurity measures the degree or probability of a particular variable being wrongly classified when it is randomly chosen. The degree of Gini index varies between 0 and 1, where 0 denotes that all elements belong to a certain class or if there exists only one class, and 1 denotes that the elements are randomly distributed across various classes. The formula of the Gini index is given in Eqn. (9.1):

$$\mathcal{G}_i = 1 - \sum_{k=1}^{k} Pik^2 \tag{9.1}$$

2. Entropy or information gain is used to determine which feature/attribute gives us the maximum information about a class. It is based on the concept of entropy, which is the degree of uncertainty,

impurity, or disorder. It aims to reduce the level of entropy starting from the root node to the leave nodes. Entropy can be found by Eqn. (9.2):

$$\mathcal{H}_i = -\sum_{k=1}^{k} Pik \log(Pik) \tag{9.2}$$

The DT algorithm tries and attempts to minimize a cost function J in Eqn. (9.3).

$$J_{(t,tk)} = \frac{M_{left} \times \mathcal{G}_{left}}{M} + \frac{M_{right} \times \mathcal{G}_{right}}{M} \tag{9.3}$$

In the above equation, M_{left} and M_{right} are a number of instances in the left node and right node after a random split of data from any particular attribute instance. G left and right is the Gini index of that node and M is a total no of instances.

The value of (k, t_k) which gives the lowest value of cost function J is taken as the root node and the second minimum value is taken as the child node and this process is repeated until the given depth and predictions are reached.

The computational complexity of the DT algorithm is given in Eqn. (9.4):

$$\Theta \log(m \times n) \tag{9.4}$$

The DT algorithm gives very good results on even large datasets with high accuracy. The nature of the DT algorithm is to overfit the data. If the depth of the tree is not provided DT algorithm will try to make the tree for every attribute and result. It is just like memorizing the whole dataset. This is not a good case as any minute change in the dataset will affect the tree structure and its predictions. In Figure 9.1, there is a general description of tree structure formed using the above method. In this general structure root node, consist of the lowest entropy or Gini cost function from here the decision is made to the second-lowest-cost function node on the left or right. This process continues until the prediction decision.

9.3.2 SUPPORT VECTOR MACHINE (SVM)

SVM is a very complex working algorithm [14]. In the SVM algorithm, there is an assumption that the data must be linearly separable as described in Figure 9.2. SVM cannot be applied to non-linearly separable data but by using Kernel with SVM, this can be applied on non-linearly separable. The SVM algorithm can only work with small and simple datasets. Its implicit working makes it appropriate for binary classification related problems. SVM is essentially based on the algorithm called maximal margin classifier. The SVM algorithm finds the best-suited hyperplane which can separate the data into two perfects domains. The points that are closest to the hyperplane are support vectors.

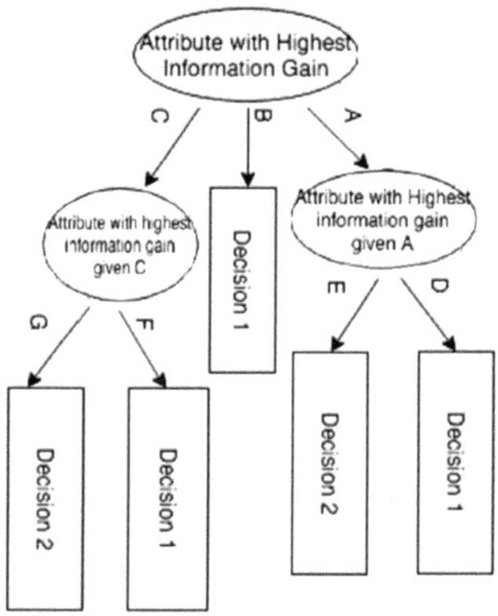

FIGURE 9.1 A general decision tree structure.

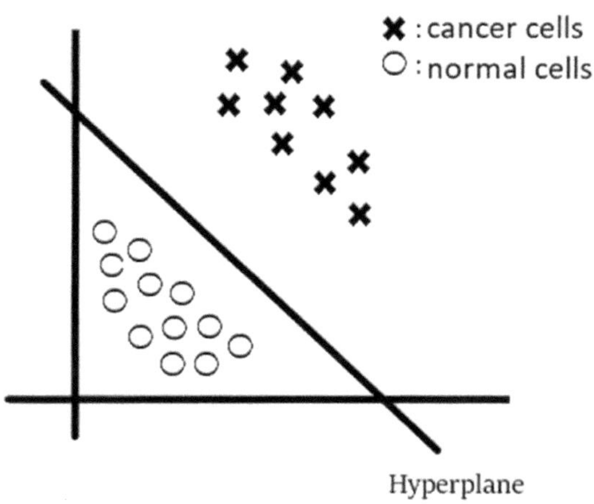

FIGURE 9.2 Linearly separable data.

In a 2D space, a hyperplane is a line, which can be represented as the Eqn. (9.5) where β are coefficients and X is a variable matrix if Eqn. (9.6) satisfies Eqn. (9.5) then 'X' lies on the hyperplane. In p dimension space, a hyperplane is represented as the Eqn. (9.7). Now when a data matrix of $n \times p$ order is defined, the hyperplane becomes as Eqn. (9.8). And when a binary classifier is defined as Eqn. (9.9), then from Eqn. (9.7) a new set of Eqns. (9.8) and (9.9) are obtained. From both Eqns. (9.8) and (9.9), it can be inferred as a compact Eqn. (9.10).

For any new observation, the SVM algorithm monitors the sign of the Eqns. (9.10)/(9.11) on the basis of which it can provide predictors.

$$\beta_0 + \beta_1 X_1 + \beta_2 X_2 = 0 \tag{9.5}$$

$$X = (X_1 X_2)^T \tag{9.6}$$

$$\beta_0 + \beta_1 X_1 + \beta_2 X_2 + \ldots + \beta_p X_p = 0 \tag{9.7}$$

$$\beta_0 + \beta_1 X_{i1} + \beta_2 X_{i2} + \ldots + \beta_p X_{ip} = 0 \tag{9.8}$$

$$y \in \{+1, -1\} \tag{9.9}$$

$$\beta_0 + \beta_1 X_{i1} + \ldots + \beta_p X_{ip} \geq 0 \; for \; y_i = +1 \tag{9.10}$$

$$\beta_0 + \beta_1 X_{i1} + \ldots + \beta_p X_{ip} < 0 \; for \; y_i = -1 \tag{9.11}$$

$$y_i(\beta_0 + \beta_1 X_{i1} + \ldots + \beta_p X_{ip}) > 0 \tag{9.12}$$

The magnitude can be thought of as the distance from the hyperplane, Where W^T are weights of an instance distance and W_0 is an arbitrary weight constant as mention in Eqns. (9.13) and (9.14). On subtracting Eqn. (9.14) from Eqn. (9.13), Eqn. (9.15) is obtained which is normalized as shown in Eqn. (9.16). This normalized equation is used as a marginal equation. The SVM algorithm attempts to maximize the margin described in Eqn. (9.14) under the constraint that no training data must be misclassified which is defined in Eqns. (9.17) and (9.18).

$$W_0 + W^T X_{positive} = +1 \tag{9.13}$$

$$W_0 + W^T X_{negative} = -1 \tag{9.14}$$

$$W^T \left(X_{positive} - X_{negative} \right) = 2 \tag{9.15}$$

$$\frac{W^T\left(X_{positive}-X_{negative}\right)}{W}=\frac{2}{W} \quad (9.16)$$

$$W_0+W^T X_{(i)}\geq 1\, for\, y_i=+1 \quad (9.17)$$

$$W_0+W^T X_{(i)}<1\, for\, y_i=-1 \quad (9.18)$$

Kernel Support Vector Machine (Kernel SVM) is similar to the SVM algorithm but before the application of SVM, SVM Algorithm uses a Kernel Trick to transform a non-linearly separable dataset into a linearly separable one. In the kernel, SVM a non-linearly separable data of P dimension is increased to the P + 1 dimension. SVM chooses a similarity function to create new coordinates for the original dataset. The most preferred Kernel is the Gaussian radial basis function (RBF) Kernel.

Gaussian RBF which is defined by Eqn. (9.19).

$$\phi\gamma(x)=\exp(-\gamma|x-l|^2) \quad (9.19)$$

where, l = landmark, and γ = separation parameter (0.3). After this, the data can be divided by hyperplane and SVM can be applied easily on the dataset. As discussed above the SVM is only suitable for small datasets due to its high complexity SVM can't be applied on a dataset with more than a large number of instances. Though it is perfect for a small dataset and where the dataset is marginally spaced and where the dataset is of high dimensions. In Figure 9.3, it can be visualized that the data separated by hyperplane and support vectors which help in SVM for classification.

9.3.3 K NEAREST NEIGHBORS (KNN)

KNN algorithm can be said as the simplest ML algorithm. It is a deterministic instance-based classification algorithm [15]. The KNN attempts to find the K nearest neighbors with respect to the test observation. The preferred distance metric is Euclidean distance. After finding the nearest neighbors KNN algorithm, the value of K in KNN must be carefully and experimentally chosen.

The space and time complexity of the KNN algorithm is tremendously large and grows in proportion with the number of observations (m) and a number of attributes (n). It is because for every new observation KNN first finds distance from every observation then sort the distances to find the nearest neighbors to classify the new point. The computational efficiency of KNN is very good. The KNN algorithm is only suitable for small and simple datasets. Figure 9.4 describes the working of the KNN algorithm in a generalized manner.

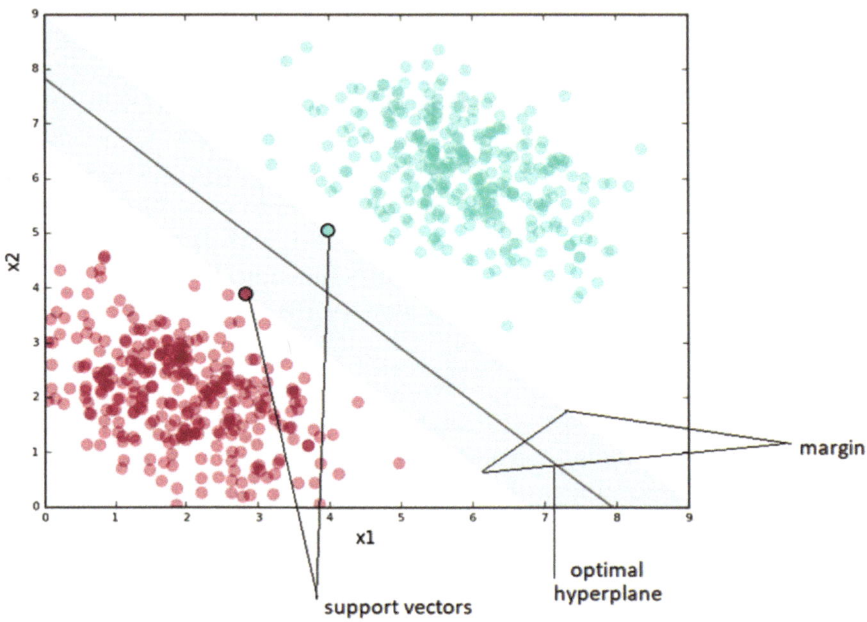

FIGURE 9.3 Graph of dataset showing support vectors and hyperplane created by SVM.

9.4 CASE STUDY AND EMPIRICAL EVALUATION OF MACHINE LEARNING (ML) ALGORITHMS

In this section, the above studied algorithms are applied to breast cancer datasets to find an algorithm with the best results. First, a brief description of the dataset is provided then an individual algorithm is applied on the dataset hence respective results are provided.

9.4.1 CASE STUDY DATASET DESCRIPTION

The breast cancer dataset has been taken for the application of ML algorithms. Dataset is available at the UCI ML repository and also inbuilt in sci-kit learn library breast cancer [16, 17]. The dataset is a multivariate dataset with no missing values it contains 32 attributes and 569 instances or observations where feature matrices contain 30 attributes which are divided as a set of 3 for mean, error, and worst of ten real-valued features computed for each cell nucleus:

1. Radius (mean of distances from the center to points on the perimeter);
2. Texture (standard deviation of gray-scale values);
3. Perimeter;
4. Area;
5. Smoothness (local variation in radius lengths);
6. Compactness (perimeter^2/area – 1.0);
7. Concavity (severity of concave portions of the contour);
8. Concave points (number of concave portions of the contour);
9. Symmetry;
10. Fractal dimension ("coastline approximation" – 1).

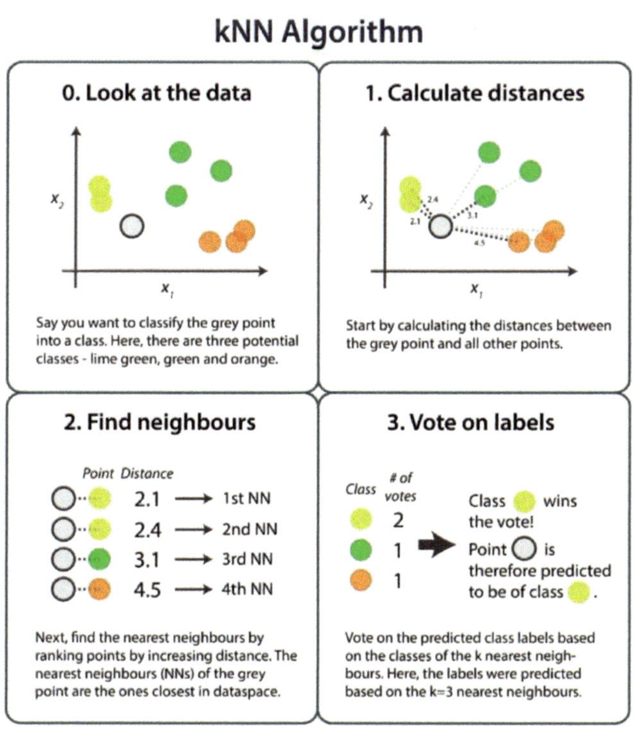

FIGURE 9.4 Working of KNN algorithm.

While two attributes are patient id and diagnosis (M = malignant, B = benign) attribute or column has been set as a vector of observations y.

Then data is preprocessed where y is encoded and X is feature scaled. Since there will be no new set of values to test the algorithm, a dataset has been divided into a training set and test set, now the algorithm is applied on the training set to find the relations and when the test set feature matrix is fed, predicted vector of observations of the test set is getting as the outcome. This split is of 0.3 or 1/3 of the dataset will be test set.

To observe the accuracy of algorithm comparison of a given vector of observation with a predicted vector of observations is done and a confusion matric is formed which is divided as:

1. true-positive;
2. true-negative;
3. false-positive; and
4. false-negative.

Where positive and negative represent two classes in binary classification. True represents where the prediction of the model and actual observation is the same, that is, the model predicted positive or negative, and actual values were also positive or negative, respectively. False represents where the model predicted positive or negative but real values were negative or positive respectively. After the successful application of all three algorithms on the dataset, their results are provided in further subsections.

9.4.2 DECISION TREE (DT) RESULTS

After applying the DT algorithm on the training set, that is, X-test, and y-test a tree structure is formed which can be visualized using the Graphviz module of the sci-kit learn library.

For every new feature in the test set, the tree is traversed and prediction is made, from Figure 9.5 it can be clearly seen that if the depth of a tree is increased better prediction can be made as it will have a greater number of features to traverse with.

The maximum depth was set as 12 but in only 8 depth level the training data was overfitted. The accuracy of the DT was 0.9476 on the test set while 0.9834 on the whole dataset.

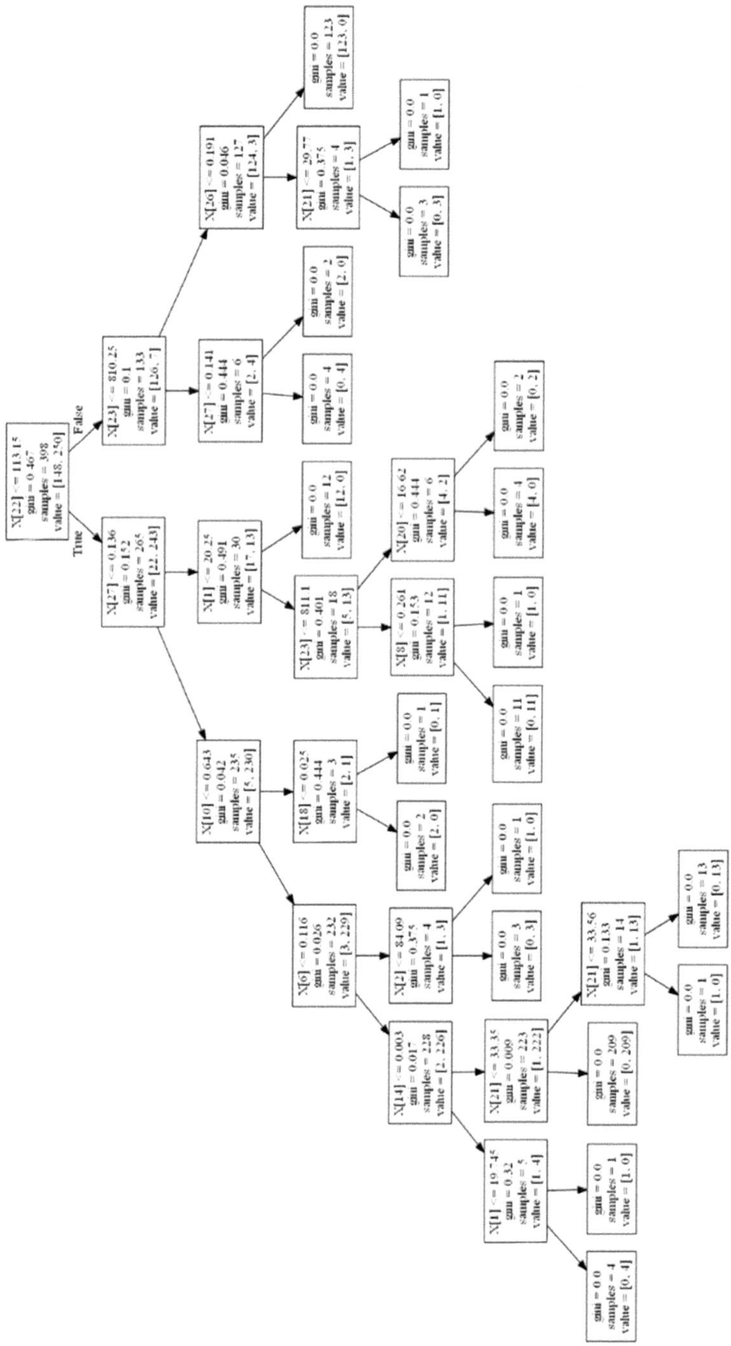

FIGURE 9.5 The decision tree on breast cancer dataset.

9.4.3 SUPPORT VECTOR MACHINE (SVM) RESULTS

On applying SVM classifier on test set accuracy of 0.6417 was obtained and 0.8840 on the whole dataset. Since it is a model-based technique, SVM is applied one time on training data and it can classify test data with the help of support vectors created in training data. But a slight change in training data can result in a change in support vector and the hyperplane created earlier can misclassify the test data that's why its accuracy is low.

9.4.4 K-NEAREST NEIGHBORS RESULTS

Applying KNN on a training set and test set yields to good results of 0.9415 accuracy level on the test set and 0.9402 on the whole dataset. There is not much difference in both results as the KNN algorithm is instance-based, that is, it will calculate the nearest neighbor for every new feature matrix value and classify it accordingly.

9.4.5 DISCUSSION

After a successful study of the results of all three algorithms, it was found that the DT algorithm gives the best results among the three. It is due to its overfitting nature where it tries to remember the whole dataset which can also be a negative aspect; if it gives 100%, accuracy there is a further method of tuning and adjusting the algorithms. Since this dataset accuracy was around 98% it can work here accurately. Hence using this algorithm an application is built which can be useful in biomedical science.

9.5 HEALTH CARE CHATBOT

The healthcare chatbot system is a GUI-based window software developed on python language and the inter-library for GUI. In this window application first, a login page appears where the user can login or register. After a successful login a new application window appears with clear, start, yes, and no buttons and two display windows as shown in Figure 9.6.

On starting the application, in question box, series of questions will be asked on whether they have the following symptoms or not to which

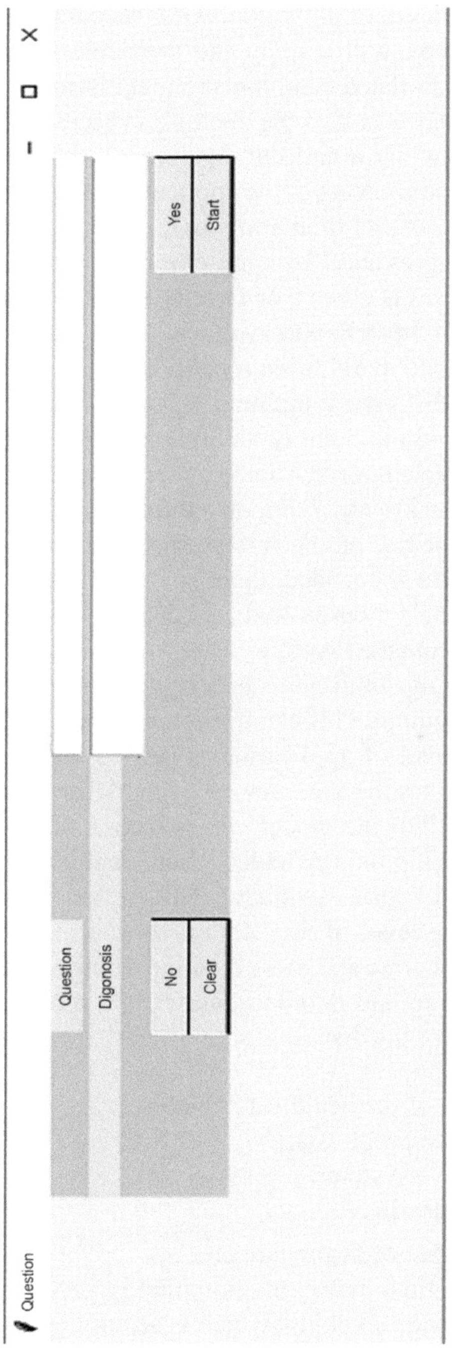

FIGURE 9.6 Application window of healthcare chatbot.

user can reply with a yes or no button. After successful questions, a series diagnosis display box will display the predicted disease by model its confidence level and related symptoms to that disease.

It will also display a link to the doctor on practo.com for consultancy. Users can clear the window and start again or close the application.

In the background working of the application, there are training and test data set for symptoms and their prognosis. Training set containing 4990 observations or diseases and 136 symptoms or features. For every disease, the value of symptoms is given 0 or 1 value on given symptoms are related to that disease or not. In 4990 observations, diseases are repeated related to symptom value 1 so to avoid these repetitions there is compression of the same disease with different symptoms. After that, the diseases have been encoded and to avoid the dummy variable trap, the encoded diseases are converted into a sparse matrix. This is a preprocessing part.

Now applying the DT algorithm on a training set to create the tree, once the tree is created, the tree has been traversed from user answer of yes or no also since all the data is encoded, there is a need to decode the data while traversing to get a final output as predicted disease. Also, the doctor's dataset has been scrapped from the Practo website where with every disease there is a link to a particular doctor. Again, applying DT on the whole doctor dataset to give a link as an output. This can be seen in Figure 9.7.

The accuracy level of application is 0.9810 on the dataset provided where accuracy defines the accuracy of the model according to the dataset. The confidence level of the model ranges from 0.08 to 0.32 according to disease given and symptoms provided where confidence level defines how confident the model is that users have that particular predicted disease or not. The confidence level of application can be increased if the dataset provided is more accurate and more detailed. If the model can be provided with a more accurate and detailed dataset, the model can have a more accurate prognosis of the disease.

- Advantages of the healthcare chatbot:
    1. Advance prognosis;
    2. Adaptive system;
    3. User friendly.
- Disadvantages of healthcare chatbot:
    1. No real-time data extraction, that is, predefined dataset.
    2. Confidence level low which is according to the dataset.

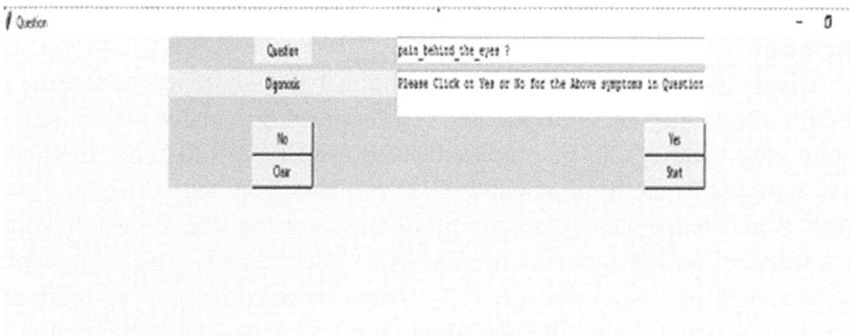


```
increased_appetite ?

yes
['You may have Diabetes ']

symptoms present  ['increased_appetite']

symptoms given ['fatigue', 'weight_loss', 'restlessness', 'lethargy',
'irregular_sugar_level', 'blurred_and_distorted_vision', 'obesity',
'excessive_hunger', 'increased_appetite', 'polyuria']

 The model suggests:

 Consult  ['Dr. Anshul Gupta']

 Visit  ['https://www.practo.com/delhi/doctor/dr-anshul-gupta-ear-nose-
 throat-ent-specialist-1?specialization=Ear-Nose-Throat%20(ENT)
 %20Specialist&practice_id=712546']
```

FIGURE 9.7 Symptoms questions and output of the diagnosis window.

9.6 CONCLUSION

In this chapter, concepts and working of a few ML algorithms have been described and their application on breast cancer data set was carried out. From this, it concludes that ML implementation in biomedical research can be very beneficial and of the three studied algorithms, DT gave the best result on the breast cancer dataset.

On applying, the same algorithm to create a healthcare chatbot and it was found that algorithm accuracy was high but changing the dataset can provide better results of prognosis. Even though this healthcare chatbot system can be very future proving application for better diagnosis and healthcare.

After studying ML in the biomedical field, it can assure its advancement in the future, since by applying ML results of breast cancer dataset and a health care chatbot can be prepared if the use of deep learning methods is an increase in the biomedical field. It can benefit in very advanced and difficult problems such as prediction of cancer using image visualization of cells, advanced prognosis and diagnosis system which can alert patients or doctors, drug discovery, etc. [19]. It can be possible as deep learning uses neural networks for the determination of results [18, 20]. Hence, it can benefit human-level intelligence with the fast processing of computer systems in the biomedical field.

KEYWORDS

- **decision tree**
- **health care chatbot**
- **K-nearest neighbors**
- **machine learning**
- **machine-learning algorithms**
- **support vector machine**

REFERENCES

1. Samuel, A. L., (1967). Some studies in machine learning using the game of checkers. II-recent progress. *IBM Journal of Research and Development, 11*(6), 601–617.
2. Mitchell, T. M., (1999). Machine learning and data mining. *Communications of the ACM, 42*(11).
3. Larranaga, P., Calvo, B., Santana, R., Bielza, C., Galdiano, J., Inza, I., & Robles, V., (2006). Machine learning in bioinformatics. *Briefings in Bioinformatics, 7*(1), 86–112.
4. Olson, R. S., La Cava, W., Mustahsan, Z., Varik, A., & Moore, J. H., (2017). *Data-Driven Advice for Applying Machine Learning to Bioinformatics Problems.* arXiv preprint arXiv:1708.05070.
5. Kotsiantis, S. B., Zaharakis, I., &Pintelas, P., (2007). Supervised machine learning: A review of classification techniques. *Emerging Artificial Intelligence Applications in Computer Engineering, 160*, 3–24.

6. Jiao, Y., & Du, P., (2016). Performance measures in evaluating machine learning based bioinformatics predictors for classifications. *Quantitative Biology*, *4*(4), 320–330.
7. Barlow, H. B., (1989). Unsupervised learning. *Neural Computation*, *1*(3), 295–311.
8. Chapelle, O., Scholkopf, B., & Zien, A., (2009). Semi-supervised learning. In: Chapelle, O., et al., (eds.), (2006) [book reviews]. *IEEE Transactions on Neural Networks*, *20*(3), 542–542.
9. Kaelbling, L. P., Littman, M. L., & Moore, A. W., (1996). Reinforcement learning: A survey. *Journal of Artificial Intelligence Research*, *4*, 237–285.
10. Aha, D. W., Kibler, D., & Albert, M. K., (1991). Instance-based learning algorithms. *Machine Learning*, *6*(1), 37–66.
11. Bishop, C. M., (2013). Model-based machine learning. *Philosophical Transactions of the Royal Society A: Mathematical, Physical, and Engineering Sciences*, *371*(1984), 20120222.
12. Kotsiantis, S. B., Kanellopoulos, D., & Pintelas, P. E., (2006). Data preprocessing for supervised leaning. *International Journal of Computer Science*, *1*(2), 111–117.
13. Friedl, M. A., & Brodley, C. E., (1997). Decision tree classification of land cover from remotely sensed data. *Remote Sensing of Environment*, *61*(3), 399–409.
14. Amari, S. I., & Wu, S., (1999). Improving support vector machine classifiers by modifying kernel functions. *Neural Networks*, *12*(6), 783–789.
15. Dudani, S. A., (1976). The distance-weighted k-nearest-neighbor rule. *IEEE Transactions on Systems, Man, and Cybernetics*, (4), 325–327.
16. Mangasarian, O. L., & Wolberg, W. H., (1990). Cancer diagnosis via linear programming. *SIAM News, 23*(5), 1 & 18.
17. William, H. W., & Mangasarian, O. L., (1990). Multi surface method of pattern separation for medical diagnosis applied to breast cytology. *Proceedings of the National Academy of Sciences, U.S.A., 87*, 9193–9196.
18. Lan, K., Wang, D. T., Fong, S., Liu, L. S., Wong, K. K., & Dey, N., (2018). A survey of data mining and deep learning in bioinformatics. *Journal of Medical Systems, 42*(8), 139.
19. Lavecchia, A., (2015). Machine-learning approaches in drug discovery: Methods and applications. *Drug Discovery Today, 20*(3), 318–331.
20. Min, S., Lee, B., & Yoon, S., (2017). Deep learning in bioinformatics. *Briefings in Bioinformatics*, *18*(5), 851–869.
21. Gupta, R., Khari, M., Gupta, D., & Crespo, R. G., (2020). Fingerprint image enhancement and reconstruction using the orientation and phase reconstruction. *Information Sciences.*
22. Khari, M., Garg, A. K., Crespo, R. G., & Verdú, E., (2019). Gesture Recognition of RGB and RGB-D Static Images Using Convolutional Neural Networks. *International Journal of Interactive Multimedia & Artificial Intelligence*, *5*(7).

CHAPTER 10

Biomedical Antennas for Medical Telemetry Applications

SARITA AHLAWAT and GARIMA SRIVASTAVA

Ambedkar Institute of Advanced Communication Technologies and Research, Delhi–110031, India,
E-mail: saritaahlawat4@gmail.com (S. Ahlawat)

ABSTRACT

In this chapter, you will learn about various antennas used in biomedical applications. Wireless biotelemetry systems operating in the radio-frequency bands are attaining a great amount of attention due to their well-enabled applications in the areas of healthcare systems inside a hospital, home, or external environments as well. In earlier times, there was wired communication of the medical devices to outside monitoring/control equipment, which majorly affected patient comfort and convenience. Therefore, biotelemetry devices with a wireless mode of communication seem to be a good solution towards improving the patients' living conditions with constant availability, well awareness of context, etc. At the present time, RF associated medical telemetry systems are additionally supported by the fast changes in wireless communications capabilities of medical devices in, on, or around the body. Antennas integrated into wireless medical devices can be divided into three categories with respect to their positioning on the patient's body: on-body antennas; implantable antennas; and ingestible antennas. These antennas are holding a very important place in biomedical applications and their use is expanding fast to meet up the requirements of wireless medical devices. Therefore, these antennas are going to gain tremendous growth in future biomedical applications providing desirable performance.

10.1 INTRODUCTION

Wireless biomedical telemetry is becoming a very promising option in health care systems as it allows a high degree of comfort for a patient to be monitored regularly and remotely. Antennas play a major role in biomedical telemetry systems to make it possible to use different wireless medical devices.

Antennas integrated into wireless medical devices can be divided into three categories with respect to their location on or inside the patient's body:

1. **On-Body Antennas:** These are positioned on the human body or worn as part of clothing. Primarily, designing antennas is carried out and integrated into medical devices which are finally positioned on the human body. Secondly, these antennas are designed to constitute part of an individual's clothing which additionally facilitates the functionalities of everyday clothing. There are different on-body medical devices such as temperature monitors, accelerometers, etc.
2. **Implantable Antennas:** These are attached to an implant and buried inside the human body to retrieve useful information. The depth of implantation plays a significant role in the performance of the antenna. Millions of people across the world are dependent on implantable medical devices to gain support and improvement in their living style. Medical implants are used widely in different applications like pacemakers, stimulators, retinal implants, etc. With a rapid increase in the growth of technologies, it is expected to see an amazing increase in their use across the world.
3. **Ingestible Antennas:** These are mostly integrated into medical devices that have the shape of a capsule to be taken as regular pills and transmit images outside of the patient's body for further diagnosing process. Wireless capsule endoscopy gains significant interest in the GI tract medical treatment. In this, the capsule is to be swallowed which sends images and video out of the body for further health monitoring. Wireless communication by ingested capsules will be done in real-time during its movement along the GI tract.

The main aim of on-body, implantable, and ingestible devices is to provide significant improvement in the living style of the patient by continuous and comfortable health monitoring systems. With the recent advancements in integration methodologies and information and communication technologies (ICTs), there is a wide scope of meaningful developments in designing and integration of miniature medical devices that can be placed in, on, or around a patient's body disallowing any form of discomfort.

10.2 ESSENTIALS OF ANTENNAS

An antenna act as the transducer which converts an electrical signal into electromagnetic (EM) energy waves and vice versa at the interface between free space and transmitting/receiving systems. Also, it can be used to optimize the radiation efficiency in some directions and minimize it in others.

There are various parameters used to describe the performance of the antenna:

- An *antenna radiation pattern* is defined as a mathematical function or a graphical representation of the radiation properties of the antenna as a function of space coordinates. It may include radiation field intensity, radiation field density, power flux, etc. Usually, the radiation pattern is determined in the far-field region and is represented as a function of the directional coordinates.
- The field format around an antenna comprises of three regions. The first region, the *reactive near-field region,* is a region where reactive field components are mainly present and it exists at a distance $R < 0.62\sqrt{D^3/\lambda}$, where λ is the wavelength, and D is the largest dimension of the radiator. The second region, the *radiating near-field (Fresnel) region,* is the field region where radiation field components are mainly present and in this region, distance from the antenna affects the angular field distribution of the antenna. The periphery of this region can be seen with $R < 2D^2/\lambda$. The third region, the *far-field (Fraunhofer) region,* the region where the distance from the antenna has not any effect on the angular field distribution of the antenna and it extends at distances larger than $2D^2/\lambda$ from the antenna. It is shown in Figure 10.1.

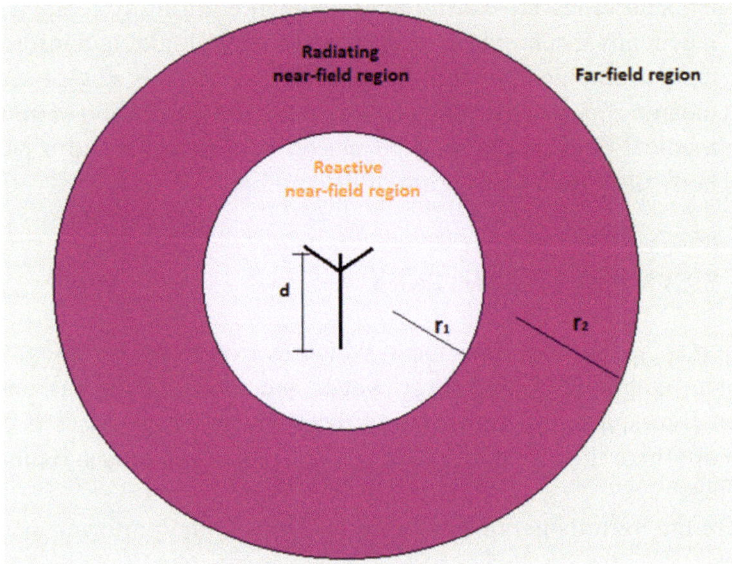

FIGURE 10.1 Field format around an antenna sub-divided into three regions.

- **Directivity:** It is the ratio of the radiation intensity in a given direction from the antenna to the radiation intensity averaged over all directions.
- **Input Impedance:** It can be defined as the ratio of the voltage to current at a pair of terminals defined as input impedance. Also, the ratio of the electric field component to the magnetic field component at a point is defined as input impedance.
- **Reflection Coefficient:** It can be defined as the ratio of the amplitude of the reflected waves to the amplitude of the incident wave. It basically shows how efficiently the transmitted power is being transferred to the antenna acting as a load in the transmitting system.

$$\text{RL} = -20\log|\Gamma|\,(dB)$$

$$\text{Where } |\Gamma| \text{ is} = \frac{V_o^-}{V_o^+} = \frac{Z_L - Z_o}{Z_L + Z_o}$$

$\Gamma|$ is the reflection coefficient

V_o^+ is the incident voltage

- **Bandwidth:** It is the number of frequencies adjacent to center frequency within which antenna performance parameters like input impedance, reflection coefficient, etc., confirm an acceptable standard value of that at the center frequency.

10.3 ON-BODY ANTENNAS

10.3.1 ANTENNA DESIGN

The design of on-body antennas needs to take care of several parameters which are summarized below. On-body antennas are gaining a growing interest in academia as well as industry; different efforts have been reported in the literature regarding the design and communication capabilities of on-body antennas to communicate with exterior monitoring/controlling equipment or even other on-body antennas.

1. **Defined Frequencies of Operation:** The Federal Communications Commission (FCC) is a regulatory authority that has allocated 608–614, 1395–1400, and 1427–1432 MHz ranges of frequencies for wireless medical telemetry service (WMTS) area and 902–928 and 2400.0–2483.5 MHz ranges of frequencies for industrial, scientific, and medical (ISM) applications in the United States. Also, the Electronic Communications Committee (ECC) has assigned the frequency bands of 433.1–434.8 and 868.0–868.6 MH for ISM applications in Europe.
2. **Antennas and Properties of Material:** On-body antennas are basically placed on the human body to assist in wireless healthcare systems. Commonly, patch and loop antennas are chosen for on-body communication applications as they offer very good conformability and flexibility in shape and size. On the other hand, monopole antennas ($\lambda/4$ length) situated on a small-sized ground plane has delivered a better performance for different on-body links and for several body postures. This performance becomes achievable as the radiation pattern of the monopole antenna is an omnidirectional that makes it more suitable for the cases where the characteristics of the wireless link are unknown. In some medical applications where directive planar inverted-F antenna (PIFA) geometries selected in order to have synchronization of the direction of maximum radiation

to the receiving antenna to obtain a significant reduction in losses in the wireless communication link while comparing to the monopole antennas. The tapered slot antenna (TSA) uses two diverging tapered slots to achieve more desirable impedance matching within the range of frequencies from 3.1 to 10.6 GHz as compared to that conventional wideband CPW-fed antenna [1]. Here, the TSA antenna depicted less group delay deviation because of weak resonance characteristics within the operating band. Additionally, its radiation pattern appeared to be more appropriate which makes it less sensitive to fluctuations in the surrounding environment.

An antenna to be implanted should be easy to attach to the human body or clothing, when it is considered in terms of material compatibility. These antennas don't suffer difficulty in integration with medical devices in terms of the material when used in on-body communication systems. Even though these antennas are relatively inexpensive, still such antennas may not be flexible and high profile. Therefore, textile antennas which are easy to be attached in the daily used individual garment are considered. There are electro textiles (e-textiles) that are able to function as electronics and at the same time physically behaving as textiles that assist the fabrication of textile antennas [2]. Both electrical properties (e.g., the conductivity of material) and mechanical properties (e.g., the flexibility of material) are very important in the fabrication process of e-textiles. The methods that are most commonly used to integrate conductivity into textiles are stitching, weaving, knitting, and printing. To get more detail, a UWB antenna [3] made from textile materials has been given at the end of the chapter. The antenna was a "fully textile" antenna as textiles were used for both substrate and conducting parts. One of the major disadvantages of most planar textile antennas proposed in the literature is that they need a coaxial cable connecting the transceiver [4].

Such a feeding method is rigid, and, thus, relatively uncomfortable to the patient wearing the antenna. To overcome such difficulties with feeding methods, a microstrip feed line structure can be preferred over the coaxial feeding technique, which allows the coupling of its power into the antenna via an aperture in the bottom ground plane. The first aperture-coupled patch antenna (ACPA) using textile materials has been given at the end of the chapter showing the enhancement in efficiency using the aperture coupling method in Hertleer et al. [5].

3. **Influence of Human Body:** The function of on-body antennas is dependent on its proximity to human tissues. There are some common issues such as detuning of an antenna, alteration in radiation pattern, and decrease in the radiation efficiency which have been discussed in detail in Refs. [6–8]. To get a clear idea of the interaction between on-body antennas and the human tissues, it brings investigation on the performance of such antennas once they are situated close to the human body.

   For biomedical applications, antennas must be immune to frequency detuning. So, wide-band antenna designs attract high attention for on-body antennas. It is to be noted that the design of an Ultra-Wide Band antenna is determined by its characteristic of the coefficient of reflection (S_{11}) as well as its capability to sustain the pulse shape, unlike its narrow-band counterpart. Therefore, UWB antenna systems should contain broader impedance bandwidth with stable and high efficiency.

   Then, some on-body antennas can be designed using electromagnetic bandgap (EBG) substrates to reduce significantly the amount of the radiation absorption within the human body and obtain desirable antenna gain and this can be understood in detail in Refs. [9, 10] given at the end of the chapter.

4. **Antenna Diversity:** The high date rate communication in continuous monitoring health care systems demands the use of multiple antennas. Hence, a technique (antenna diversity) where more than two signals from several independent antennas are mixed in different ways to form a unique signal is becoming a more attractive option. This technique can be employed in different ways. It can be implemented with the deployment of different antennas, that is, space diversity, different patterns of radiation characteristics, that is, pattern diversity, or different types of polarization, that is, polarization diversity. Space diversity is obtained by using multiple antennas at the transmitter or receiver side. This technique can be understood more deeply in Ref. [11] given at the end of the chapter. Pattern diversity is one of the diverse techniques that can be achieved by using different radiation patterns in the one or separate radiator. Finally, polarization diversity is also one of the diverse techniques

that can be achieved through a single antenna with more than one polarization or different antennas with different polarizations.

The main purpose behind the incorporation of the antenna diversity technique is to minimize channel fading problem and enable an efficient channel link in terms of power transfer. Here, the problem of fading can probably arise because of the mobile nature of the human body parts, polarization mismatch, and scattering within the heterogeneous body structure and surrounding environment in the case of on-body channels. The use of diversity prevents deep fades. The improvement seen through the diversity technique is most commonly quantified in terms of the diversity gain (DG).

10.3.2 CHANNEL MODELING

There are two possible communication channels suggested to provide communication with on-body medical devices:

1. **On-Body Channels:** These are used to provide the wireless mode of communication between on-body medical devices/components on the body in wireless medical systems. They consist of transmission paths on the human body and also paths scattering off the local environment of the body (indoors or outdoors).
2. **Off-Body Channels:** These are used to provide the wireless mode of communication between an on-body medical device and an exterior controlling device and deal with EM wave propagation around the human body.

For instance, on-body medical devices can communicate with a wearable device using both on- and off-body propagation channels in the case of a biomedical telemetry application. In this case, the wearable device may act as a controller that passes data between the on-body devices and remote stations.

Wave propagation in on-body and off-body channels is more complicated as compared to propagation between two antennas in free space, for example, between a cellular phone and a cellular base station. Firstly, the dynamic nature of the human body is prominent. In normal activities, movements of the human body can be significant or, in certain cases (e.g., sports), extreme. The human body is subject to several small movements' case even while standing or sitting. Thus, the characteristics of the wireless link and system performance suffer fluctuations.

Furthermore, the numerical computation related to the human body is complex as attributed to variations in anatomy and dielectric properties between individuals as well as varying dielectric properties of tissues with frequency. The need for accurate simulation of the body's postures and movements is also highly challenging. Hence, it becomes necessary to develop deterministic and generic channel models in order to enable the design of reliable and robust communication links for on-body medical devices.

10.4 IMPLANTABLE ANTENNAS

10.4.1 ANTENNA DESIGN

The implantable antenna is one of the very popular antennas integrated with medical devices used for continuous health monitoring. It is really important to consider some factors like selection of operation frequency, biocompatibility, electronics, and power consumption while designing an implantable antenna.

1. **Selection of Operation Frequency:** The International Telecommunications Union–Radio communications Recommendation SA-1346 [12] allocated the frequency band from 402 MHz to 405 MHz for Medical Implant Communications Systems (MICS) for in-body communication. There is also another frequency band 2400–2500 MHz for ISM communication systems. These frequency bands are chosen based upon the placement and position of the antenna on the human body related to the required capabilities of communication.
2. **Type and Material of Antenna:** The selection of type and material of antenna require significant attention in wireless biotelemetry systems. The implantation of the antenna must be biocompatible in order to maintain the safety level of patients under monitoring. Mostly, patch designs are preferred considering their flexibility and conformability in design. In addition, the human body has large inhomogeneous characteristics because of the different properties of skin tissue, muscle, and fat. These variations in surrounding materials inside the human body considerably impact the performance of antenna as the implanted antennas may come in direct contact with surrounding material causing a short circuit of metallization. Therefore, another dielectric layer is placed for preserving

the required biocompatibility of the antenna as well as separating the conducting radiator (Figure 10.2). There are some commonly used biocompatible materials like Teflon having permittivity, MACOR, and ceramic alumina. Encasing the desired antenna by a thin layer of biocompatible material is an alternate method to achieve biocompatibility in antenna designing (Figure 10.2b).

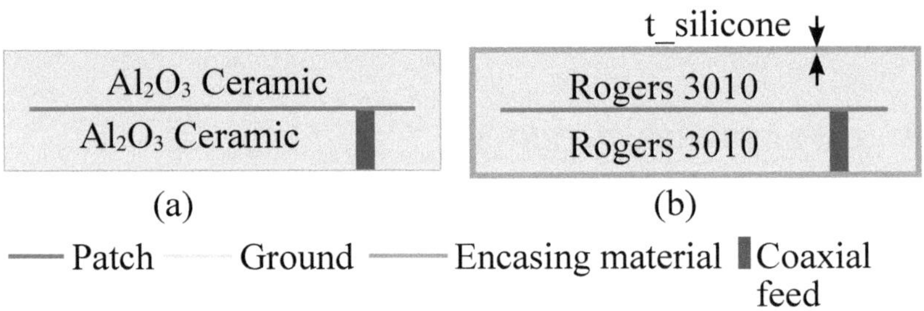

FIGURE 10.2 Two approaches to address the biocompatibility issue for practical applications: (a) proposed antenna with biocompatible material and (b) proposed antenna with encased biocompatible material [72].

3. **Miniaturization:** It is the most important factor while designing implantable antennas for wireless medical telemetry systems. This is very much desirable for in-body communication applications like glucose monitoring where continuous monitoring is performed.

There are several techniques to achieve miniaturization of the implantable antenna while designing for in, on, or around body communications as below:

1. **Use of Dielectric Substrate/Superstrate having high Dielectric Constant:** The high-permittivity dielectric substrate/superstrate is the most commonly used method to compress the size of the implantable radiator. This high-permittivity of substrate/superstrate reduces the effective wavelength which brings the resonant frequency to a lower frequency value. The commonly used ones are Rogers RO3210/RO3010/6002, having a relative dielectric constant of 10.2.
2. **Increment in the Path of Flowing Current Over the Radiator:** Another approach has meandered/spiraled line/slot incorporation to gain a considerable reduction of size. As the path of current flowing over the surface of the radiator increases, the frequency of resonance shifts to a lower frequency value which results in size reduction.

3. **Incorporation of Reactive Loads for Impedance Matching:** Impedance matching can be obtained by using the loading method. For example, in the link given here https://doi.org/10.1007/s41870-018-00276-5, capacitive loading provides an antenna size compression of a considerable amount by using the proposed antenna design. Shorting pins between the radiating patch structure and the ground plane can provide considerable shortening in the size of the antenna.
4. **Higher Operating Frequency:** Several ranges of higher frequencies have been allocated to gain miniaturization operation for the required application at hand. Additionally, higher operating frequency allows a wider bandwidth of communication for high data-rate communication. But at the same time, high operating frequency suffers from large losses due to biological tissues in the human body. Consequently, this trade-off between size reduction and losses due to surrounding material should be taken into account carefully to set requirements under monitoring.
5. **Patient Safety Considerations:** Patient safety is the utmost requirement of any healthcare system. This parameter is monitored by the amount of power incident to the implantable antenna being dissipated per unit of mass. The specific absorption rate (SAR) is the most commonly used parameter to measure the rate of energy deposited per unit mass of tissue and ensuring to meet standard international guidelines related to patient safety issues. This SAR depicts electric field intensity distribution due to the implantable antenna inside the human body. Two SAR limitations (1.6 W/kg per 1-g averaging and 2 W/kg for 10-g averaging) must be followed carefully under transmission from an implantable device. The geometry and compositions of the body play an important role in the accurate computation of field intensities and consequently accurate SAR measurement.

Peak SAR is defined as:

$$\text{SAR}\ (r_0) = \frac{1}{2}\frac{\sigma_e'(r_0)\left|\text{E}(r_0)\right|^2}{\rho(r_0)}$$

where, r_o is the point of measurement, σ_e is the electrical conductivity of surrounding material, ρ is the mass density of the medium, and $\frac{1}{2}\sigma'_e|E|^2$ is the absorbed power density (averaged) at the point of measurement, r_0.

10.4.2 CHANNEL MODELING

Modeling of the biomedical telemetry channel for implantable antennas is one of the challenging parts of biotelemetry systems. Unlike the propagation in free-space, propagation within a heterogeneous human body is quite different and lossy due to their diverse electrical characteristics. Hence, it becomes important to model the channel considering the refraction, diffraction, reflection, and absorption of EM field propagating within the body.

10.5 INGESTIBLE ANTENNAS

The patient faces significant discomfort in the conventional methods which are used to treat disorders related to the GI tract. Therefore, it is gaining the high attention of researchers to develop ingestible antennas that can be integrated into a capsule and swallowed for an examination of the entire digestive tract.

10.5.1 ANTENNA DESIGN

1. **Selection of Operation Frequency:** The scientific community takes significant attention while selecting an operating frequency for ingestible antennas. For example, the efficiency of an antenna can be enhanced by increasing frequency. On the other side, higher frequencies may cause an increase in radiation absorption due to the presence of the body tissues. Furthermore, this may degrade the performance of the communication link and demanding more supply powers that posing questions regarding the safety of the patient.

   In 2003a [15], an ingestible antenna within the human body has a considerable impact of surrounding material within the body inside the frequency range of 150.00 MHz–1.20 GHz, which is detailed here. Significant radiation was present within a range of frequencies from 450 to 900 MHz and field intensity out of the body exhibited distribution similar to a Gaussian distribution. Even though in this reference, the operating range of frequencies is from 434.0 MHz to 915.0 MHz of the ISM bands, these bands are not appropriate for digital video transmission. On the other side, there is a better-developed transmission of video signals in the 2.450 GHz frequency band for WLAN and Bluetooth applications (technologically), antennas/radiators, camera modules, and other RF electronic components. In the end, high frequencies of transmission considerably reduce the size of antennas and electronic components resulting in the effective integration of ingestible devices in medical applications. Hence, the 2.45 GHz band appears to be a good promising solution. For example, an IC design for wireless capsule endoscopy at 2.4 GHz has been discussed in Ref. [16] given at the end of the chapter.

2. **Type and Material of Antenna:** It is very important to make stable and accurate health monitoring in wireless-capsule endoscopic systems. To retrieve accurate and real-time information from wireless capsule endoscopy, ingestible antennas must exhibit omnidirectional radiation pattern and circular polarization to minimize the sensitivity in terms of orientation as compared to implantable antennas. As the swallowed capsule moves along the GI tract, its exact position and alignment are not generally known. Hence, an isotropic radiation field pattern is desirable for ingestible antennas in biomedical domains.

   Taking the above considerations, normal mode helical antennas are most commonly used for such applications. As wireless capsule endoscope systems, need to transmit real-time and high-resolution data hence miniaturized and wide bandwidth antenna are required here. For example, a wideband spiral antenna has been presented in detail at 500 MHz for ingestible capsule endoscope systems in Ref. [17] given at the end of the chapter.

   Although the FDTD method has the ability to model anatomically detailed human body structures in corresponding geometries, there are still many challenges in modeling small size antennas. Like implantable antennas, ingestible antennas must also be biocompatible to maintain the quality of a patient's life. These requirements entail assembling of the ingestible antenna, sensors, camera, and other electronic components inside a shell. It is found that capsule casings and circuitry have a negligible effect on the ingestible antenna performance.

3. **Patient Safety Considerations:** Safety guidelines in the designing of an ingestible antenna at high frequencies require significant attention. Two parameters such as SAR and rise in temperature of ingestible antennas have been discussed to show the performance

of antenna at frequencies ranging from 430.0 MHz to 3.0 GHz in Ref. [18] given at the end of the chapter. Results depicted that high values of SAR and temperature rise were observed near the location of the ingestible device.

4. **Positioning and Directional Considerations:** Ingestible antenna depicts different performances for various locations inside the body and their antenna orientations. These positioning and orientation effects have been discussed in detail in Ref. [15] where Numerical investigations using the FDTD method have been performed for a male human subject and an ingestible monofilar helix antenna having dimensions as 8 mm diameter, 4 mm length, and pitch of 1 mm. The range of frequencies was starting from 150 MHz up to a frequency of 1.2 GHz. Near and far-field results exhibited the radiation intensity was maximum experienced on the anterior side of the human body. Furthermore, there was no direct correlation between the near and far-fields. Vertically polarized waves had to suffer attenuation than its counterpart. Thus, their performance can be improved by making proper antenna orientation in a designated band of operation.

10.5.2 CHANNEL MODELING

The modeling of the channel between the integrated ingestible antenna of a medical device and an exterior antenna of exterior monitoring/control device requires high attention to get desirable performance.

Considering far-field communication, the link power budget can be described in terms of:

$$\begin{aligned}\text{Link margin (dB)} &= \text{Link } C/N_0 - \text{Required } C/N_0 \\ &= P_t + G_t - L_f + G_r - N_0 \\ &\quad - E_b/N_0 - 10\log_{10} B_r + G_c - G_d\end{aligned}$$

where, P_t is the power of transmitting antenna, G_t is the gain of transmitting antenna, G_r is the gain of receiving antenna, L_f is the path loss (in free space), and N_o is the noise power spectral density.

According to the degradation in strength of the signal as it travels along the length of separation between the transmitting and receiving antenna in free space signal strength, the path loss can be found as below:

$$L_f(\text{dB}) = 20\log\left(\frac{4\pi d}{\lambda}\right)$$

where, d is the length of separation between the transmitting and receiving antenna. Consider the impedance mismatch loss:

$$L_{\text{imp}}(\text{dB}) = -10\log\left(1-|\Gamma|^2\right)$$

where, Γ is the appropriate reflection coefficient. Also:

$$\alpha = \text{Re}(\gamma) = \text{Re}\left(j\omega\sqrt{\mu\varepsilon}\sqrt{1-j\frac{\sigma}{\omega\varepsilon}}\right)$$

E and σ are the permittivity and conductivity values of the medium at an angular frequency of w, respectively.

The above equations can be used to evaluate communication link performance inside the human body taking into consideration the corresponding heterogeneous structure of the surrounding material. As the values of conductivity and permittivity will be highly dependent on the different human body tissues while the signal is propagating out of the human body.

10.6 CONCLUSION AND FUTURE SCOPE OF DIRECTIONS

Antennas are the very important component in wireless medical systems for biomedical applications. Depending on the antenna, designing and positioning, antennas have been classified into three types of antennas such as on-body, implantable, and ingestible antennas. Research efforts made in the field of antenna designing and channel modeling have provided good confidence to incorporate these antennas in various medical applications. New research directions can also be incorporated for further optimization.

On-body antennas facilitate bidirectional communication with exterior equipment. In on-body antennas, research can be continued on textile antennas and e-textile materials to make their transmission more reliable in terms of washable packaging of the electronics, durable interconnections, and long-term behavior. Metamaterials can be used to reduce surface currents which in turn minimize the antenna-to-body coupling and improving the communication link performance of the antennas.

Implantable antennas are the most widely used antennas in the biotelemetry systems. In an earlier time, inductive communication links were found very popular to make communication possible used to provide communication between the devices. But, these communication links had disadvantages like a short range of communication capability, low data rate, and high patient's discomfort. Thus, wireless medical systems based on RF links appear to be a better solution in biotelemetry applications. Remote monitoring systems allow the distant diagnosis and treatment of diseases and reduce the hospitalization period. Electrically small antennas exhibit low radiation distribution and narrow bandwidth. So, the design of multiband antennas is also significant for harvesting energy and increasing the lifetime of the device. The implantable antenna designing and performance analysis can be further taken into considerations with the use of more efficient simulation tools and human body tissue models. The experimental testing in terms of measurements within living animals is very intriguing and requires careful consideration to create an efficient testing protocol.

Ingestible antennas are gaining high interest in the scientific community to make diagnosing of GI tract more reliable and efficient. In ingestible antennas, research efforts can be considered further in determining the relation between radiation characteristics, antenna position, and orientation. There are some uncertainties that need to be taken into accounts such as the placement of the arms, which may influence the near field, or the existence of clothing, which may affect the temperature rise. Studies regarding the wireless communication link of ingestible antennas can be done to a larger extent as EM wave propagation in free space has given in this chapter as a foundation of the wireless propagation phenomenon.

KEYWORDS

- **axial ratio (AR) bandwidth**
- **circular polarization**
- **implantable antenna**
- **industrial scientific and medical band**
- **ingestible antenna**
- **microstrip patch antenna**
- **miniaturization**
- **radio frequency (RF)**

REFERENCES

1. Chen, Z. N., (2005). Novel bi-arm rolled monopole for UWB applications. *IEEE Trans. Antennas Propag., 53*(2), 672–677.
2. Klemm, M., Locher, I., & Tröster, G., (2004). A novel circularly polarized textile antenna for wearable applications. In: 7th *Europ Microw Week* (pp. 137–140). Amsterdam, the Netherlands.
3. Osman, M. A. R., Rahim, M. K. A., Samsuri, N. A., Salim, H. A. M., & Ali, M. F., (2011). Embroidered fully textile wearable antenna for medical monitoring applications. *Prog. Electrom. Res., 117*, 321–337.
4. Tronquo, A., Rogier, H., Hertleer, C., & Van, L. L., (2006). A robust planar textile antenna for wireless body plans operating in the 2.45-GHz ISM band. *Inst. Elect. Eng. Electron. Lett., 42*(3), 142–143.
5. Hertleer, C., Tronquo, A., Rogier, H., Vallozzi, L., & Van, L. L., (2007). Aperture-coupled patch antenna for integration into wearable textile systems. *IEEE Antennas Wireless Propag. Lett., 6*, 392–395.
6. Scanlon, W. G., & Evans, N. E., (2001). Numerical analysis of body worn UHF antenna systems. *IEE Electron Commun. Eng. J., 13*(2), 53–64.
7. Okoniewski, M., & Stuchly, M. A., (1996). A study of the handset antenna and human body interaction. *IEEE Trans. Microw. Theory Tech., 44*(10), 1855–1864.
8. Wong, K. L., & Lin, C. I., (2005). Characteristics of a 2.4-GHz compact shorted patch antenna in close proximity to a lossy medium. *Microw. Opt. Technol. Lett., 45*(6), 480–483.
9. Salonen, P. O., Yang, F., Rahmat-Samii, Y., & Kivikoski, M., (2004a). WEBGA-Wearable electromagnetic band-gap antenna. *IEEE Antennas Propag. Int. Symp., 1*, 451–454.
10. Zhu, S., & Langley, R., (2009). Dual-band wearable textile antenna on an EBG substrate. *IEEE Trans. Antennas Propag., 57*(4), 926–935.
11. Khan, I., Hall, P. S., Serra, A. A., Guraliuc, A. R., & Nepa, P., (2009). Diversity performance analysis for on-body communication channels at 2.45 GHz. *IEEE Trans. Antennas Propag., 57*(4), 956–963.
12. International Telecommunications Union-Radio Communications (ITU-R), (1998). *Recommendation ITU-R SA.1346.*
13. Karacolak, T., Cooper, R., & Topsakal, E., (2009). Electrical properties of rat skin and design of implantable antennas for medical wireless telemetry. *IEEE Trans. Antennas Propag., 57*(9), 2806–2812.
14. Karacolak, T., Cooper, R., Butler, J., Fisher, S., & Topsakal, E., (2010). In vivo verification of implantable antennas using rats as model animals. *IEEE Antennas Wireless Propag. Lett., 9*, 334–337.
15. Chirwa, L. C., Hammond, P. A., Roy, S., & Cumming, D. R. S., (2003a). Electromagnetic radiation from ingested sources in the human intestine between 150 MHz and 1.2 GHz. *IEEE Trans. Biomed. Eng., 50*, 484–492.
16. Xie, X., Li, G., Chen, X. K., Li, X. W., Chi, B. Y., & Han, S. G., (2004). A novel low power IC design for bi-directional digital wireless endoscopy capsule system. *IEEE Int. Workshop Biomed. Circuit. Syst.*, 185–188.

17. Lee, S. H., Lee, J., Yoon, Y. J., Park, S., Cheon, C., Kim, K., & Nam, S., (2011). A wideband spiral antenna for ingestible capsule endoscope systems: Experimental results in a human phantom and a pig. *IEEE Trans. Biomed. Eng., 58*(6), 1734–1741.
18. Xu, L., Maz, M. Q. H., Ren, H., & Chan, Y., (2008b). Radiation characteristics of ingested wireless device at frequencies from 430 MHz to 3 GHz. *IEEE Conf. Eng. Med. Biol. Soc.,* 1250–1253.
19. Abadia, K., Merli, F., Zurcher, J. F., Mosig, J. R., & Skrivervik, A. K., (2009). 3D Spiral small antenna design and realization for biomedical telemetry in the MICS band. *Radio Engineering, 18*(4), 359–367.
20. Abbasi, Q. H., Alomainy, A., & Hao, Y., (2011b). Characterization of MB-OFDM-based ultra-wideband systems for body-centric wireless communications. *IEEE Antennas Wireless Propag. Lett., 10,* 1401–1404.
21. Abbasi, Q. H., Sani, A., Alomainy, A., & Hao, Y., (2010). On-body radio channel characterization and system-level modeling for multiband OFDM ultra-wideband body-centric wireless network. *IEEE Trans. Microw. Theory Tech., 58*(12), 3485–3492.
22. Abbasi, Q. H., Sani, A., Alomainy, A., & Hao, Y., (2011a). Experimental characterization and statistical analysis of the pseudo dynamic ultra-wideband on-body radio channel. *IEEE Antennas Wireless Propag. Lett., 10,* 748–751.
23. Ahlawat, S., Srivastava, G., & Kumar, G., (2019). *Int. J. Inf. Tecnol.* https://doi.org/10.1007/s41870-018-00276-5 (accessed on 29 July 2020).
24. Alomainy, A., & Hao, Y., (2009). Modeling and characterization of biotelemetric radio channel from ingested implants considering organ contents. *IEEE Trans. Antennas Propag., 57,* 999–1005.
25. Alomainy, A., Hao, Y., & Pasveer, F., (2007a). Numerical and experimental evaluation of a compact sensor antenna for healthcare devices. *IEEE Trans. Biomed. Circ. Syst., 1*(4), 242–249.
26. Alomainy, A., Hao, Y., Owadally, A., Parini, C. G., Nechayev, Y., Constantinou, C. C., & Hall, P. S., (2007b). Statistical analysis and performance evaluation for on-body radio propagation with microstrip patch antennas. *IEEE Trans. Antennas Propag., 55*(1), 245–248.
27. Alomainy, A., Hao, Y., Parini, C. G., & Hall, P. S., (2005). Comparison between two different antennas for UWB on-body propagation measurements. *IEEE Antennas Wireless Propag. Lett., 4,* 31–34.
28. Alomainy, A., Sani, A., Rahman, A., Santas, J. G., & Hao, Y., (2009). Transient characteristics of wearable antennas and radio propagation channels for ultra-wideband body-centric wireless communications. *IEEE Trans. Antennas Propag., 57*(4), 875–884.
29. Attiya, A. M., & Safaai-Jazi, A., (2004). Simulation of ultra-wideband indoor propagation. *Microw. Opt. Technol. Lett.*, 42(2), 103–108.
30. Balanis, C. A., (2002). *Antenna Theory: Analysis and Design* (2nd edn.). New York: Wiley.
31. Chan, Y., Meng, M. H., Wu, K. L., & Wang, X., (2005). Experimental study of radiation efficiency from an ingested source inside a human body model. *IEEE Eng. Med. Biol. Soc.*, 7754–7757.
32. Chen, Z. N., (2007). *Antennas for Portable Devices.* New York: Wiley.

33. Chirwa, L. C., Hammond, P. A., Roy, S., Cumming, D. R. S., (2003b). Radiation from ingested wireless devices in biomedical telemetry bands. *IEEE Electron. Lett., 39*(2), 178–179.
34. Conway, G. A., & Scanlon, W. G., (2009). Antennas for over-body-surface communication at 2.45 GHz. *IEEE Trans. Antennas Propag., 57*(4), 844–855.
35. Fort, A., Desset, C., Ryckaert, J., De Doncker, P., Van, B. L., & Donnay, S., (2005). Ultra-wide-band body area channel model. *IEEE Int. Conf. Commun., 4*, 2840–2844.
36. Gemio, J., Parron, J., & Soler, J., (2010). Human body effects on implantable antennas for ISM bands applications: Models comparison and propagation losses study. *Prog. Electrom. Res., 110*, 437–452.
37. Hall, P. S., Hao, Y., Nechayev, Y. I., Alomainy, A., Constantinou, C. C., Parini, C., Kamarudin, M. R., et al., (2007). Antennas and propagation for on-body communication systems. *IEEE Antennas Propag. Mag., 49*(3), 41–58.
38. Hu, Z. H., Nechayev, Y. I., Hall, P. S., Constantinou, C. C., & Hao, Y., (2007). Measurements and statistical analysis of on-body channel fading at 2.45 GHz. *IEEE Antennas Wireless Propag. Lett., 6*, 612–615.
39. Institute of Electrical and Electronics Engineers (IEEE), (1999). IEEE standard for safety levels with respect to human exposure to radiofrequency electromagnetic fields, 3 kHz to 300 GHz. *IEEE Standard C95.1-1999.*
40. Institute of Electrical and Electronics Engineers (IEEE), (2005). IEEE standard for safety levels with respect to human exposure to radiofrequency electromagnetic fields, 3 kHz to 300 GHz. *IEEE Standard C95.1-2005.*
41. International Commission on Non-Ionizing Radiation Protection (ICNIRP), (1998). Guidelines for limiting exposure to time-varying electric, magnetic, and electromagnetic fields (up to 300 GHz). *Health Phys., 74*, 494–522.
42. Jovanov, E., O'Donnell-Lords, A., Raskovic, D., Cox, P., Adhami, R., & Andrasik, F., (2003). Stress monitoring using a distributed wireless intelligent sensor system. *IEEE Eng. Med. Biol. Mag., 22*(3), 49–55.
43. Kawoos, U., Tofighi, M. R., Warty, R., Kralick, F. A., & Rosen, A., (2008). *In-vitro* and *in-vivo* trans-scalp evaluation of an intracranial pressure implant at 2.4 GHz. *IEEE Trans. Microw. Theory Tech., 56*(10), 2356–2365.
44. Khan, I., & Hall, P. S., (2009). Multiple antenna reception at 5.8 and 10 GHz for body-centric wireless communication channels. *IEEE Trans. Antennas Propag., 57* (1), 248–255.
45. Kim, J., & Rahmat-Samii, Y., (2004). Implanted antennas inside a human body: Simulations, designs, and characterizations. *IEEE Trans. Microw. Theory Techn., 52*(8), 1934–1943.
46. Kim, J., & Rahmat-Samii, Y., (2006). SAR reduction of implanted planar inverted F antennas with non-uniform width radiator. *IEEE Int. Symp. Antennas Propag.*, 1091–1094.
47. Kiourti, A., & Nikita, K. S., (2011). Meandered versus spiral novel miniature PIFAs implanted in the human head: Tuning and performance. In: *2nd ICST Int. Conf. Wireless Mobile Commun. Healthcare* (pp. 80–87). Kos Island, Greece.
48. Kiourti, A., & Nikita, K. S., (2012a). A review of implantable patch antennas for biomedical telemetry: Challenges and solutions. *IEEE Antennas Propag. Mag., 54*(3), 210–228.

49. Kiourti, A., & Nikita, K. S., (2012b). Miniature scalp-implantable antennas for telemetry in the MICS and ISM bands: Design, safety considerations and link budget analysis. *IEEE Trans. Antennas Propag., 60*(6), 3568–3575.
50. Kiourti, A., & Nikita, K. S., (2012c). Accelerated design of optimized implantable antennas for medical telemetry. *IEEE Antennas Wireless Propag. Lett., 11*, 1655–1658.
51. Kiourti, A., & Nikita, K. S., (2012d). Recent advances in implantable antennas for medical telemetry. *IEEE Antennas Propag. Mag., 54*(6), 190–199.
52. Kiourti, A., & Nikita, K. S., (2013). Design of implantable antennas for medical telemetry: Dependence upon operation frequency, tissue anatomy and implantation site. *Int. J. Monit. Surv. Technol., 1*(1), 16–33.
53. Kiourti, A., Christopoulou, M., & Nikita, K. S., (2011). Performance of a novel miniature antenna implanted in the human head for wireless biotelemetry. *IEEE Int. Symp. Antennas Propag.* (pp. 392–395). Spokane, Washington.
54. Kiourti, A., Psathas, K. A., Costa, J. R., Fernandes, C. A., & Nikita, K. S., (2013). Dual-band implantable antennas for medical telemetry: A fast design methodology and validation for intra-cranial pressure monitoring. *Prog. Electrom. Res., 141*, 161–183.
55. Lee, C. M., Yo, T. C., Huang, F. J., & Luo, C. H., (2009). Bandwidth enhancement of planar inverted-F antenna for implantable biotelemetry. *Microw. Opt. Technol. Lett., 51*(3), 749–752.
56. Liu, W. C., Chen, S. H., & Wu, C. M., (2008). Implantable broadband circular stacked PIFA antenna for biotelemetry communication. *J. Electromagn. Waves Appl., 22*, 1791–1800.
57. Liu, W. C., Chen, S. H., & Wu, C. M., (2009). Bandwidth enhancement and size reduction of an implantable PIFA antenna for biotelemetry devices. *Microw. Opt. Technol. Lett., 51*(3), 755–757.
58. Rajagopalan, H., & Rahmat-Samii, Y., (2010). Link budget analysis and characterization for ingestible capsule antenna. *Int. Workshop Antenna Technol.*, 1–4.
59. Rucker, D., Al-Alawi, A., Adada, R., & Al-Rizzo, H. M., (2007). A miniaturized tunable micro strip antenna for wireless communications with implanted medical devices. *ICST 2nd Int. Conf. on Body Area Networks* (pp. 1–4). Brussels, Belgium.
60. Salonen, P., Rahmat-Samii, Y., Hurme, H., & Kivikoski, M., (2004b). Dual band wearable textile antenna. *IEEE Antennas Propag. Soc. Int. Symp.*, 463–466.
61. Sani, A., Rajab, M., Foster, R., & Hao, Y., (2010). Antennas and propagation of implanted RFIDs for pervasive healthcare applications. *Proc. IEEE, 98*(9), 1648–1655.
62. Serra, A. A., Nepa, P., Manara, G., & Hall, P. S., (2007). Diversity measurements for on-body communication systems. *IEEE Antenna Wireless Propag. Lett., 6*(1), 361–363.
63. Soontornpipit, P., Furse, C. M., & Chung, Y. C., (2004). Design of implantable micro strip antenna for communication with medical implants. *IEEE Trans. Microw. Theory Tech., 52*, 1944–1951.
64. Soontornpipit, P., Furse, C. M., & Chung, Y. C., (2005). Miniaturized biocompatible microstrip antenna using genetic algorithm. *IEEE Trans. Antennas Propag., 53*(6), 1939–1945.
65. Valdastri, P., Menciassi, A., Arena, A., Caccamo, C., & Dario, P., (2004). An implantable telemetry platform system for *in vivo* monitoring of physiological parameters. *IEEE Trans. Inf. Technol. Biomed., 8*(3), 271–278.

66. Wang, Q., & Wang, J., (2009). Performance of on-body chest-to-waist UWB communication link. *IEEE Microw. Wireless Compon. Lett.*, *19*(2), 119–121.
67. Warty, R., Tofighi, M. R., Kawoos, U., & Rosen, A., (2008). Characterization of implantable antennas for intracranial pressure monitoring: Reflection by and transmission through a scalp phantom. *IEEE Trans. Microw. Theory Tech.*, *56*(10), 2366–2376.
68. Xia, W., Saito, K., Takahashi, M., & Ito, K., (2009). Performances of an implanted cavity slot antenna embedded in the human arm. *IEEE Trans. Antennas Propag.*, *57*(4), 894–899.
69. Xu, L., Max, Q. H., & Ren, H. L., (2008a). Electromagnetic radiation from ingested sources in the human intestine at the frequency of 2.4 GHz. *Progress Electrom. Res. Symp.*, 893–897.
70. Xu, L., Meng, M. Q. H., & Chan, Y., (2009a). Effects of dielectric parameters of human body on radiation characteristics of ingestible wireless device at operating frequency of 430 MHz. *IEEE Trans. Biomed. Eng.*, *56*, 2083–2094.
71. Xu, L., Meng, M. Q. H., Ren, H., & Chan, Y., (2009b). Radiation characteristics of ingestible wireless devices in human intestine following radiofrequency exposure at 430, 800, 1200, and 2400 MHz. *IEEE Trans Antennas Propag.*, *57*, 2418–2428.

Index

G

H

I

J

K

L

T

X

Y

Z